LIVING THERAPY

D0861668

Counselling for Eating Disorders in Women

Person-Centred Dialogues

Richard Bryant-Jefferies

Radcliffe Publishing

Oxford • Seattle

Radcliffe Publishing Ltd
18 Marcham Road
Abingdon
Oxon OX14 1AA
United Kingdom

www.radcliffe-oxford.com
Electronic catalogue and worldwide online ordering facility.

British Library Cataloguing in Publication Data

A catalogue record for this book is available from the British Library.

ISBN 1 85775 776 9

Typeset by Aarontype Ltd, Easton, Bristol
Printed and bound by TJ International Ltd, Padstow, Cornwall

Contents

Foreword

I am delighted to have been asked to contribute to this excellent and innovative book, even though I have no certainty about the protocol of writing something such as a foreword. It is a real privilege because this book will be particularly helpful to other person-centred counsellors such as myself, who are working in the field of eating disorders.

Having become acquainted with Richard's writing through his earlier work in the *Living Therapy* series on *Counselling Young People* and *Problem Drinking*, I value not only his style of writing but also his presentation of the person-centred approach in practice. As a lecturer in counselling I have many times referred my students to Richard's work as a way of seeing the approach in action.

In my work both as a counsellor and supervisor I recognise the importance of a book such as this one, as I believe it fills a gap in the eating disorders literature that has existed for a long time. Much of the literature is either from a psychodynamic or a cognitive behavioural perspective which leaves those of us who are person-centred counsellors struggling to understand the complexity of the client who has an eating disorder, without the benefit of literature to support our work. Although there may be those who will argue that the person-centred approach is person specific rather than problem specific, nonetheless many clients describe their experience in problem specific terms. It was this gap in the literature that drove me recently to carry out a small-scale study on eating disorders and I presented my findings within the context of the person-centred approach, many of which are supported throughout this book.

The strengths of the book are in my opinion two-fold: the ease with which Richard is able to demonstrate how the theory of the person-centred approach can aid our understanding of a client with an eating disorder and how he can explain the potential process of change for someone with an eating disorder; second, I have been impressed by the depth of relationship that Richard is able to convey through the different sessions, even though the sessions themselves are fictitious, which feel powerful enough for the reader to be able to enter the experience as a 'fly on the wall' and very swiftly have an experiential understanding of the session.

This I believe also means that the book lends itself not only to counsellors and students of counselling but to other professionals of whom there are often many involved in the care of clients who have an eating disorder. A wish of mine is that the emphasis Richard places on the supervisory relationship is picked up and responded to positively by those professionals outside the counselling profession. As with my own work within this field supervision has been vitally important in understanding not only my client but my own process within the relationship.

Richard demonstrates a capacity to enter the world of clients who have an eating disorder in a very powerful and creative way, his words at times have moved me especially at those points where he illuminated an aspect of the work that I feel is crucial for clients such as these, for example the struggle to know they exist. This is a beautifully crafted and thought provoking book — a real gift.

Lorna Marchant
Senior Lecturer
University of Brighton
Counsellor, supervisor, trainer and consultant
September 2005

Foreword

This is the first of Richard Bryant-Jefferies' books that I have read, and I am pleased to become acquainted with his innovative portrayal of a client-centered therapeutic process. His succinct summary of the approach will be valuable to readers unfamiliar with client-centered work, and the comments he embeds within the sample cases carries this learning and reflection throughout, reminding us of key choices we make as client-centered practitioners. I am particularly impressed with the clear voices of his characters and the attention to detail in the therapists' self-reflective dialogues. Richard addresses the difficult issues brought on by working with clients who have physical as well as psychological risks, but advocates throughout for a consistent, careful practice of the client-centered model. I believe he offers a valuable tool to both the beginning therapist considering this approach and to the advanced clinician expanding skills.

As a client-centered therapist practicing in the United States, I often find myself alone in describing the rationale for my clinical choices. Discussing work with clients experiencing eating and body image difficulties provides a particular challenge because I am often at odds with a clinical culture that is increasingly sure of diagnosis, medications, and manualized treatments as the most effective routes to change. Richard Bryant-Jefferies' work provides helpful arguments supporting the value and therapeutic rationale of preserving self-direction even with a client who may be behaving at odds with her best physical interests. I am supportive of a client utilizing all resources available, including medication, support groups, self-help books, other techniques, etc., especially as sought out or requested by the client. But I appreciate that Richard notes that engaging in any planned program of goal setting, recommendations, or medical interventions not requested by the client, would, without any surety of quicker or longer lasting relief, disrupt the carefully constructed healing relationship we are sure of creating as client-centered practitioners.

I am also especially pleased with the attention paid to the consultation relationship. These scenarios well illustrate a person-centered take on such choices as integrating family members into sessions or unraveling the fears we have that clients may be unaware of the physical dangers their eating behaviors may cause. I particularly resonate to the consultation scenario which shows a therapist processing her desire to take action with a bingeing client where she would likely sit more patiently with a cutting or suicidal person. This provides an interesting opportunity to reflect on the factors that may influence a therapist to fall into pushing, worrying for, or medically managing a client, even when this therapist is otherwise strongly committed to the client's right to self-direction. Richard Bryant-Jefferies offers us a chance to consider that our fears about not intervening may, with heightened awareness, be better recognized as personal discomforts with the behaviors or fears of not understanding or of participating in unknown physical damage, but are not likely to reveal appropriate or effective interventions that would cause the client to better care for herself more expediently. I agree that a client-centered therapist can respond to client need and physical distress without departing from a non-directive stance and feel that this approach remains the most likely to offer the client an opportunity to examine her struggle and find relief.

I believe that this book captures the precision needed to honor the self-direction of a client struggling with eating disorders. Richard Bryant-Jefferies shows how a client-centered practitioner incorporates appropriate responses to and care for a person who may suffer symptoms or risks as a result of her eating behaviors. I appreciate being given the opportunity to comment on this book and look forward to using this and the other *Living Therapy* books in my teaching.

Carolyn Schneider MA, LCPC
Director of Mental Health Services, Center on Halsted
Chicago, Illinois
September 2005

Preface

The success of the preceding volumes in the *Living Therapy* series, and the continued appreciative comments received from readers and by independent reviewers, is encouragement enough to once again extend this style into exploring the application of the person-centred approach to counselling and psychotherapy to another key area of difficulty within the human experience. Again and again people remark on how readable these books are, how much they bring the therapeutic process alive. In particular, students of counselling and psychotherapy have remarked on how accessible the text is. Trainers and others who are experienced in the field have indicated to me the timeliness of a series that focuses the application of the person-centred approach to working therapeutically with clients having particular issues. This is both heartening and encouraging. I want the style to draw people into the narrative and feel engaged with the characters and the therapeutic process. I want this series to be what I would term 'an experiential read'.

As with the other titles in the *Living Therapy* series, *Counselling for Eating Disorders in Women: person-centred dialogues* is composed of fictitious dialogues between fictitious clients and their counsellors, and between their counsellors and their supervisors. Within the dialogues are woven the reflective thoughts and feelings of the clients, the counsellors and the supervisors, along with boxed comments on the process and references to person-centred theory. I do not seek to provide all the answers, or a technical manual expounding on the right way to work with female clients who are experiencing an eating, or eating-related problem or set of problems. Rather I want to convey something of the process of working with representative material that can arise so that the reader may be stimulated into processing their own reactions, and reflecting on the relevance and effectiveness of the therapeutic responses, to thereby gain insight into themselves and their practice. Often it will simply lead to more questions which I hope will prove stimulating to the reader and encourage them to think through their own theoretical, philosophical and ethical positions and their boundary of competence.

Counselling for Eating Disorders in Women: person-centred dialogues is intended as much for experienced counsellors as it is for trainees. It provides real insight into what can occur during counselling sessions. I hope it will raise awareness of, and inform, not only person-centred practice within this context, but also contribute to other theoretical approaches within the world of counselling, psychotherapy, and the various branches of psychology. Reflections on the therapeutic process and points for discussion are included to stimulate further thought and debate. Included in this book is material to inform the training process of counsellors and others who seek to work with women on these issues.

So, how does the person-centred counsellor approach working with a client who is experiencing the effects of problematic eating or an eating issue that has generated a problematic health condition? I hope that this book will demonstrate the value, relevance and effectiveness of this approach, providing, as it does, a very human response to what is a very human problem. I hope that in this book I am able to address a range of themes that leave you, the reader, with much to reflect on and to take into your professional counselling work, whatever the setting.

Richard Bryant-Jefferies
September 2005

About the author

Richard Bryant-Jefferies qualified as a person-centred counsellor/therapist in 1994 and remains passionate about the application and effectiveness of the approach. Between early 1995 and mid-2003 Richard worked at a community drug and alcohol service in Surrey as an alcohol counsellor. Since 2003 he has worked for the Central and North West London Mental Health NHS Trust, managing substance misuse service within the Royal Borough of Kensington and Chelsea in London. He has experience of offering both counselling and supervision in NHS, GP and private settings, and has provided training through 'alcohol awareness and response' workshops. He also offers workshops based on the use of written dialogue as a contribution to continuing professional development and within training programmes. His website address is www.bryant-jefferies.freeserve.co.uk

Richard had his first book on a counselling theme published in 2001, *Counselling the Person Beyond the Alcohol Problem* (Jessica Kingsley Publishers), providing theoretical yet practical insights into the application of the person-centred approach within the context of the 'cycle of change' model that has been widely adopted to describe the process of change in the field of addiction. Since then he has been writing for the *Living Therapy* series, producing an on-going series of person-centred dialogues: *Problem Drinking, Time Limited Therapy in Primary Care, Counselling a Survivor of Child Sexual Abuse, Counselling a Recovering Drug User, Counselling Young People, Counselling for Progressive Disability, Relationship Counselling: sons and their mothers, Responding to a Serious Mental Health Problem, Person-Centred Counselling Supervision: personal and professional, Counselling Victims of Warfare, Workplace Counselling in the NHS, Counselling for Problem Gambling, Counselling for Eating Disorders in Men* and *Counselling for Obesity*. The series aims to bring the reader a direct experience of the counselling process, an exposure to the thoughts and feelings of both client and counsellor as they encounter each other on the therapeutic journey, and an insight into the value and importance of supervision. Richard is also writing his first novel, 'Dying to Live', a story of traumatic loss, alcohol use and the therapeutic and has also adapted one of his books as a stage or radio play, and plans to do the same to other books in the series if the first is successful. However, he is currently seeking an opportunity for it to be recorded or staged.

Richard is keen to bring the experience of the therapeutic process, from the standpoint and application of the person-centred approach, to a wider audience.

He is convinced that the principles and attitudinal values of this approach and the emphasis it places on the therapeutic relationship are key to helping people create greater authenticity in themselves and in their lives, leading to a fuller and more satisfying human experience. By writing fictional accounts to try and bring the therapeutic process alive, to help readers engage with the characters within the narrative – client, counsellor and supervisor – he hopes to take the reader on a journey into the counselling room. Whether we think of it as pulling back the curtains or opening a door, it is about enabling people to access what can and does occur within the therapeutic process.

Acknowledgements

I often read acknowledgements in other peoples' books and am struck by the number of people mentioned. I then look at my acknowledgements and they seem so short. I tend to acknowledge only those people who have, in some way, directly contributed to what I have written, or supported and encouraged me in my writing. Perhaps this is not enough? Over the years so many people – at workshops, conferences, in supervision, general discussion – have contributed to my thinking and perception, with regard to the theme of this book and to the others in the *Living Therapy* series. So, whilst I am not mentioning names, I do wish to acknowledge their presence in my life and the fact that my thinking now is the product of an on-going process of learning and development to which so many people have contributed.

More specifically, however, I would like to thank Lorna Marchant and Carolyn Schneider for the Forewords and for their encouraging words about this book. I would also like to thank the Eating Disorder Association for its permission to quote from its website.

Last, but not least, I would again like to express my appreciation to the team at Radcliffe Publishing and to my partner, Movena Lucas, with whom I am constantly sharing ideas in relation to the shape and content of these books, and who has fortunately grown to accept that when I have an idea it becomes so alive to me that I have to write it down.

Introduction

Counselling for Eating Disorders in Women: person-centred dialogues has been written with the aim of demonstrating the counsellor's application of the person-centred approach (PCA) in working with women who are experiencing problems associated with their eating patterns. This theoretical approach to counselling has the power of the relational experience. This relational experience is at the heart of effective therapy, contributing to the possibility of releasing the client to realise greater potential for authentic living. The approach is widely used by counsellors working in the UK today: in a membership survey in 2001 by the British Association for Counselling and Psychotherapy, 35.6% of those responding claimed to work to the PCA, whilst 25.4% identified themselves as psychodynamic practitioners. However, whatever the approach, it seems to me that the relationship is the key factor in contributing to a successful outcome – though this must remain a very subjective concept for who, other than the client, can really define what experience is to be taken as a measure of a successful outcome?

This introduction contains an overview of person-centred theory, together with a description of Rogers' ideas on the stages of psychological change and the characteristics of change within the person (*see* Appendix 1 for a list of these characteristics as Rogers described them). It also contains information about the scale and nature of eating disorders amongst women, the use of language in addressing these issues and a brief introduction to the Prochaska and DiClemente (1982) cycle of change model.

Eating disorders in women

In many respects, the notion of 'eating disorder' is one that has emerged during the latter decades of the twentieth century. Sara Gilbert (2000) points to the significance of Susie Orbach's book *Fat is a Feminist Issue* (1978), which drew attention to compulsive eating and the notion of the fear of fat in the context of women's relationships with men. The feminist movement played a key role in raising awareness of this issue, with many more books being written placing dieting and the whole issue of preoccupation with body image in the context of a sexist society. She also draws attention to the role of psychiatry in promoting a recognition of eating disorders, citing Gerald Russell (1979) who worked with people with anorexia nervosa but who also highlighted the existence of another syndrome which he called 'bulimia nervosa'.

However, eating disorders are not simply those that are diagnosed as 'anorexia nervosa' or 'bulimia nervosa'. Binge-eating and habitual heavy eating can also be considered as eating disorders. The difficulty can be where to draw the line between dieting or excessive eating to deal with life experiences and entrance into a diagnosed condition. In many cases a distorted perception of body image is also present and thus diagnosis extends beyond the eating behaviour into the realm of the psychology that drives the eating/starving pattern of behaviour.

Much has since been written exploring theories of causation and treatment of eating disorders. In general, when eating disorders are being discussed the association is with women. The young anorexic or bulimic girl, struggling to cope with maturation, and/or an idealised body shape, or to experience control over something in her life, will tend to come to mind. It may also be a way for her to deal with traumatic experiences, such as rape and sexual abuse, or extreme home situations – either excessive control and discipline or the other extreme – chaos and a lack of boundaries.

However, increasing numbers of middle-aged and older women are also developing eating disorders – some may have experienced eating disorders in early life and have lapsed into the previous eating/non-eating patterns. For others it will be a new feature in their lives. It may stem from a sense of their lives becoming out of control or unmanageable and food and weight becoming an area that they feel they can control. Thompson (1996) has pointed out that with increases in divorce, women can feel that they need to be thin to attract another partner, or that their body shape had contributed to the marriage break-up, when in fact the real reasons may have been other marital problems. Also, some women may focus more on their diet once children leave home to fill a void in their lives, believing they will perhaps feel better if they feel thin. But it is not only about dieting and weight loss, older women may gain weight through turning to food for comfort, as a way of filling a void in their lives or to handle stress.

How might we define eating disorders? The following is taken from the Eating Disorder Association website:

'Anorexia nervosa' means 'loss of appetite for nervous reasons' but this is misleading because in reality you have lost the ability to allow yourself to satisfy your appetite. You probably restrict the amount you eat and drink, sometimes to a dangerous level. You may exercise to burn off what you perceive to be excess calories. You focus on food in an attempt to cope with life, not to starve yourself to death. It is a way of demonstrating that you are in control of your body weight and shape. Ultimately, however, the disorder itself takes control and the chemical changes in the body affect the brain and distort thinking, making it almost impossible for you to make rational decisions about food. As the illness progresses, you will suffer from the exhaustion of starvation. Occasionally people die from the effects of anorexia, especially if it is untreated.

The term bulimia nervosa means literally 'the nervous hunger of an ox'. The hunger, however, is really an emotional need that cannot be satisfied by food alone. After binge-eating a large quantity of food to fill the emotional or hunger gap, there is an urge to immediately get rid of the food by vomiting or taking laxatives (or both), by starving or reducing food intake, or by working off the calories with exercise in an attempt not to gain weight.

Binge eating disorder (BED), like bulimia, has only recently been recognised as a distinct condition; it was first acknowledged as a disorder in its own right in 1992. Binge eating disorder shares some of its characteristics with bulimia but the essential difference is that you binge uncontrollably but do not purge. It is believed that many more people suffer from BED than either anorexia or bulimia nervosa. Because of the amount of food eaten, many people with BED become obese, this can lead to problems with blood pressure, heart disease and a general lack of fitness. The treatment for BED is in some ways similar to that for bulimia.

Compulsive over-eating is a variation on binge eating when you will eat at times when you are not hungry. This may happen all the time, or it may come and go in cycles. Most people who are compulsive eaters are overweight, and may use their weight or appearance as a shield they can hide behind to avoid social interaction, others hide behind a happy or jolly façade to avoid confronting their problems. Sufferers often have great shame at being unable to control the compulsion to eat. Compulsive over-eating is a serious condition and needs professional support to ensure long-term recovery.[1]

Language of eating disorders

People eat particular foods, or avoid eating for many reasons, and to the person themselves these can seem quite normal and reasonable. Even the individual who is starving themselves is doing so for a reason, however misguided that reasoning may seem to someone outside of their skin. But it is a behaviour and often an attempt, by that person, to achieve something that they desperately need. The difficulty is that so often their striving to control their diet, weight, size or shape, gets out of control, at which point it might be termed 'problematic'.

An eating disorder is an outer and visible sign of an inner condition. Unless that inner state is addressed, outer change is less likely to be sustainable. On this basis, the 'eating disorder' is secondary to the inner, psychological process that drives the behaviour. Should we therefore develop a different language that affirms this?

Perhaps we might introduce the word 'problematic' into the vocabulary when we think of eating disorders, talking instead of 'problematic or problem eating'.

---

[1] Taken from the Eating Disorder Association website: http://www.edauk.com. This is a valuable site that offers information on eating disorders and their treatments, including publications, self-help ideas and useful contacts.

The term 'eating disorder' is now largely associated in peoples' minds with females. A new language might help to widen the association in peoples' minds of this set of conditions to include both genders. It is important to note that eating disorders affect men and boys.

There is a further issue concerning language. The term eating disorder can also be regarded as 'pathologising' a particular behaviour, and causing the actual and unique underlying cause for a particular person to become lost in generalisations that are more to do with symptomatic effects and behaviours than the psychological causation. An eating disorder is, surely, a specific eating-related behaviour that has meaning for a particular person as a result of their psychological state?

It has long been said 'we are what we eat', but I would suggest reversing this as well. 'We eat what we are' captures the notion that what we eat, how we eat, how much we eat, is an expression or reflection, of the person. Do I deserve to eat healthy food, or will anything do? How much of my time will I give to preparing fresh food or is the 'fast food' solution 'good enough'? Have I a sense of needing to be full to feel good? Or is my sense of self enhanced by feeling thin? Eating style and content is expressive of the person. It becomes a disorder, arguably, when it is producing physiological damage or at risk of causing damage, or when it is associated with mental and emotional states that, for whatever reason (and usually in the person's mind there is a very good reason) are producing distortions in that person's perception of their body (body dysmorphia).

Cycle of change model

The cycle of change model was devised in the early 1980s by two American psychologists Prochaska and DiClemente (1982) and later revised (DiClemente and Prochaska, 1998). It describes the process and stages people pass through when undergoing change. It was originally devised in relation to smoking, but has been widely applied to people who have addictive behaviours – for instance, in relation to drug and alcohol use. Recently, DiClemente (2003) has produced his own book offering a more detailed description of the application of this model in treating addiction. It is an approach that has also been applied to working with patients having weight problems (Sharman, 2004). The cycle of change model suggests that people pass through stages of change and each stage has certain characteristics and demands particular areas of focus and response in order to help the client move on as listed below.

- Pre-contemplation: the client is not thinking about change.
- Contemplation: the client is beginning to think about change and/or weighing up the pro's and con's of change.
- Preparation: the client has decided to make changes and is actively preparing a plan of action.
- Action: the phase during which the planned change is put into effect.

- Maintenance: change is maintained, and if sustained the client then exits the cycle.
- Lapse or relapse: the client lapses on the planned change or returns to the original pattern.

Clients may exit the process at contemplation or at preparation if they feel that the time is not right for change, or simply find themselves unable to sustain their motivation. They may exit the cycle at maintenance having achieved their goal, whether that is a change of eating habit and/or achieving and maintaining a certain level of weight loss or weight gain. Finally, they may exit at lapse or relapse, returning to their previous pattern of eating as a result of which they may choose not to try to change, or they may return to pre-contemplation to reflect on and learn from their process so far.

What is key is to bear in mind that whilst there is change taking place in eating behaviour, this has to be underpinned by a psychological process of change. The person-centred counsellor, for instance, would not direct the client around this model; it exists to inform the process. Clients often find it interesting to have a handout so they can think for themselves what the different stages mean to them. They may see different stages, or want to use their own language to define their process. All of this is perfectly reasonable and acceptable. But the psychological process of change must not be lost sight of in the rush to achieve behaviour modification. Gradual and informed change, sustained over time, is more valuable than a cycle of constant failure which can be psychologically debilitating, and undermining of the person.

It is not within the scope of this book to consider the model further. Readers who are interested will find more information in the publications cited above.

The person-centred approach (PCA)

The PCA was formulated by Carl Rogers, and references are made to his ideas within the text of this book. However, it will be helpful for readers who are unfamiliar with this way of working to have an appreciation of its theoretical base.

Rogers proposed that certain conditions, when present within a therapeutic relationship, would enable the client to develop towards what he termed 'fuller functionality'. Over a number of years he refined these ideas, which he defined as 'the necessary and sufficient conditions for constructive personality change'. These he described as follows.

1 Two persons are in psychological contact.
2 The first, whom we shall term the client, is in a state of incongruence, being vulnerable or anxious.
3 The second person, whom we shall term the therapist, is congruent or integrated in the relationship.
4 The therapist experiences unconditional positive regard for the client.

5 The therapist experiences an empathic understanding of the client's internal frame of reference and endeavours to communicate this experience to the client.

6 The communication to the client of the therapist's empathic understanding and unconditional positive regard is to a minimal degree achieved (Rogers, 1957, p. 96).

The first necessary and sufficient condition given for constructive personality change is that of 'two persons being in psychological contact'. However, although he later published this as simply 'contact' (Rogers, 1959) it is suggested (Wyatt and Sanders, 2002, p. 6) that this was actually written in 1953–4. They quote Rogers as defining contact in the following terms: 'Two persons are in psychological contact, or have the minimum essential relationship when each makes a perceived or subceived difference in the experiential field of the other' (Rogers, 1959, p. 207). A recent exploration of the nature of psychological contact from a person-centred perspective is given by Warner (2002).

Contact

There is much to reflect on when considering a definition of 'contact' or 'psychological contact'. Is contact either present or not, or is there a kind of continuum with greater or lesser degrees of contact? It seems to me that it is both. That, rather like the way that light may be regarded as either a particle or a wave, contact may be seen as a specific state of being, or as a process, depending upon what the perceiver is seeking to measure or observe. If I am trying to observe or measure whether there is contact, then my answer will be in terms of 'yes' or 'no'. If I am seeking to determine the degree to which contact exists, then the answer will be along a continuum. In other words, from the moment of minimal contact there is contact, but that contact can then extend as more aspects of the client become present within the therapeutic relationship which, itself, may at times reach moments of increasing depth.

Empathy

Rogers defined empathy as meaning 'entering the private perceptual world of the other ... being sensitive, moment by moment, to the changing felt meanings which flow in this other person ... It means sensing meanings of which he or she is scarcely aware, but not trying to uncover totally unconscious feelings' (1980, p. 142). It is a very delicate process, and it provides a foundation block to effective person-centred therapy. The counsellor's role is primarily to establish empathic rapport and communicate empathic understanding to the client. This latter point is vital. Empathic understanding only has therapeutic value where it is communicated to the client.

There is so much more to empathy than simply letting the client know what you understand from what they have communicated. It is also, and perhaps more significantly, the actual *process* of listening to a client, of attending – facial expression, body language, and presence – that is being offered and communicated and received *at the time that the client is speaking, at the time that the client is experiencing what is present for them*. It is, for the client, the knowing that, in the moment of an experience the counsellor is present and striving to be an understanding companion.

Unconditional positive regard

Within the therapeutic relationship the counsellor seeks to maintain an attitude of unconditional positive regard towards the client and all that they disclose. This is not 'agreeing with', it is simply warm acceptance of the fact that the client is being how they need or choose to be. Rogers wrote, 'when the therapist is experiencing a positive, acceptant attitude towards whatever the client *is* at that moment, therapeutic movement or change is more likely to occur (1980, p. 116). Mearns and Thorne suggest that 'unconditional positive regard is the label given to the fundamental attitude of the person-centred counsellor towards her client. The counsellor who holds this attitude deeply values the humanity of her client and is not deflected in that valuing by any particular client behaviours. The attitude manifests itself in the counsellor's consistent acceptance of and enduring warmth towards her client' (Mearns and Thorne, 1988, p. 59).

Wilkins and Bozarth (1998) assert that 'unconditional positive regard is the curative factor in person-centred therapy' (Bozarth and Wilkins, 2001, p. vii). It is perhaps worth speculatively drawing these two statements together. We might then suggest that the unconditional positive regard experienced and conveyed by the counsellor, and received by the client, as an expression of the counsellor's valuing of their client's humanity, has a curative role in the therapeutic process. We could then add that this may be the case more specifically for those individuals who have been affected by a lack of unconditional warmth and prizing in their lives.

Congruence

Last, but by no means least, is that state of being that Rogers referred to as congruence, but which has also been described in terms of 'realness', 'transparency', 'genuineness', 'authenticity'. Indeed Rogers wrote that '... genuineness, realness or congruence ... this means that the therapist is openly being the feelings and attitudes that are flowing within at the moment ... the term transparent catches the flavour of this condition' (Rogers, 1980, p. 116). Putting this into the therapeutic setting, we can say that 'congruence is the state of being of the counsellor when her outward responses to her client consistently match the inner feelings and sensations which she has in relation to her client' (Mearns and Thorne, 1999, p. 84). Interestingly, Rogers makes the following comment in his interview with Richard Evans that with regard to the three conditions, 'first, and most important, is therapist congruence or genuineness . . . one description of what it means to be congruent in a given moment is to be aware of what's going on in your experiencing at that moment, to be acceptant towards that experience, to be able to voice it if it's appropriate, and to express it in some behavioural way' (Evans, 1975).

I would suggest that a congruent expression by the counsellor of their feelings or reactions has to emerge through the process of being in therapeutic relationship with the client. Indeed, the condition indicates that the therapist is congruent or integrated into the relationship. This indicates the significance of the relationship. Being congruent is a disciplined way of being and not an open door to endless self-disclosure. Congruent expression is perhaps most appropriate and therapeutically valuable where it is informed by the existence of an empathic understanding of the client's inner world, and is offered in a climate of a genuine warm acceptance towards the client. It is reasonable to suggest that, taking Rogers' comment quoted above regarding congruence as 'most important', we might suggest that unless the therapist is congruent in themselves and in the relationship, then their empathy and unconditional positive regard would be at risk of not being authentic or genuine.

Another view, however, would be that it is in some way false to distinguish or rather seek to separate out the three 'core conditions', that they exist together as a whole, mutually dependent on each others' presence in order to ensure that therapeutic relationship is established.

Perception

There is also the sixth condition, of which Rogers wrote: 'the final condition . . . is that the client perceives, to a minimal degree, the acceptance and empathy which the therapist experiences for him. Unless some communication of these attitudes has been achieved, then such attitudes do not exist in the relationship as far as the client is concerned, and the therapeutic process could not, by our hypothesis, be initiated' (Rogers, 1957). It is interesting that he uses the words 'minimal degree', suggesting that the client does not need to *fully* perceive the fullness of the empathy and unconditional positive regard present within, and communicated by, the counsellor. A glimpse accurately heard and empathically understood is enough to have positive, therapeutic effect although logically one might think that the more that is perceived, the greater the therapeutic impact. But if it is a matter of intensity and accuracy, then a client experiencing a vitally important fragment of their inner world being empathically understood may be more significant to them, and more therapeutically significant, than a great deal being heard less accurately and with a weaker sense of therapist understanding. The communication of the counsellor's empathy, congruence and unconditional positive regard, received by the client, creates the conditions for a process of constructive personality change.

The vital importance of contact and of the client perceiving the presence of the counsellor's unconditional positive regard and empathic understanding towards him cannot be understated. Condition numbers one and six of the necessary and sufficient conditions for constructive personality change as formulated by Rogers have become a focus for theoretical discussion and debate, and rightly so. Whilst they may not represent 'core conditions' insofar as the attitudinal qualities of empathy, congruence and unconditional positive regard are concerned, they provide the relational framework through which these attitudinal qualities can have therapeutic value and effect. Indeed, without the presence of contact and perception as described by Rogers (1957, 1959), there would be no relational framework for the therapeutic process to occur. It leaves us, perhaps, with the position that perhaps conditions one (contact) and six (perception) are in reality the 'primary core conditions' as they define the presence of a relationship. Then, unconditional positive regard and empathic understanding might be seen to define the quality of the relationship, whilst client incongruence and counsellor congruence define the state of being brought into the relationship. Taken together there emerges the existence of what we might then term as being a 'person-centred therapeutic relationship'.

Relationship is key

PCA regards the relationship that counsellors have with their clients, and the attitudes that they hold within that relationship, to be key factors. In my experience, many adult psychological difficulties develop out of life histories that involve problematic, conditional or abusive relational experiences. These can be centred in childhood or later in life. Significantly, the individual is left, through relationships that have a negative conditioning effect, with a distorted perception of themselves and their potential as a person. Patterns are established in early life, bringing their own particular problems, however they can be exacerbated by conditional and psychologically damaging experiences later in life, that in some cases will have resonance to what has occurred in the past, exacerbating the effects still further.

An oppressive experience can impact on a child's confidence in themselves, leaving them anxious, uncertain and moving towards establishing patterns of thought, feeling and behaviour associated with the developing concept of themselves typified by 'I am weak and cannot expect to be treated any differently', 'I just have to accept this attitude towards me, what can I do to change anything?' These psychological conclusions may rest on patterns of thinking and feeling already established; perhaps the person was bullied at school, or experienced rejection in the home. They may have had a life-time of stress, or it may be a relatively new experience, either way a thinking may develop typified by 'it's normal to feel stressed, you just keep going, whatever it takes'.

The result is a conditioned sense of self, with the individual thinking, feeling and acting in ways that enable them to maintain their self-beliefs and meanings within their learned or adapted concept of self. These are then lived out, the person seeking to satisfy what she has come to believe about herself: needing to care either because it has been normalised, or in order to prove to herself and the world that she is a 'good' person. She will need to maintain this conditioned sense of self and the sense of satisfaction that this gives her when it is lived out because she has developed such a strong identity with it. A particular eating pattern can be one factor in maintaining a particular sense of self, or in creating a new one in order to escape from discomfort.

The term 'conditions of worth' applies to the conditioning mentioned previously that is frequently present in childhood, and at other times in life, when a person experiences that their worth is conditional on their doing something, or behaving, in a certain way. This is usually to satisfy someone else's needs, and can be contrary to the client's own sense of what would be a satisfying experience. The values of others become a feature of the individual's structure of self. The person moves away from being true to themselves, learning instead to remain 'true' to their conditioned sense of worth. This state of being in the client is challenged by the person-centred therapist by offering them unconditional positive regard and warm acceptance. Such a therapist, by genuinely offering these therapeutic attitudes, provides the client with an opportunity to be exposed to what may be a new experience or one that in the past they have dismissed, preferring to stay with that which matches and therefore reinforces their conditioned sense of worth and sense of self.

By offering someone a non-judgemental, warm and accepting, and authentic relationship – (perhaps a kind of 'therapeutic love'?) – that person can grow into a fresh sense of self in which their potential as a person can become more fulfilled. It enables them to liberate themselves from the constraints of patterns of conditioning. Such an experience fosters an opportunity for the client to redefine themselves as they experience the presence of the therapist's congruence, empathy and unconditional positive regard. This process can take time. Often the personality change that is required to sustain a shift away from what have been termed 'conditions of worth' may require a lengthy period of therapeutic work, bearing in mind that the person may be struggling to unravel a sense of self that has been developed, sustained and reinforced for many decades of life. Of course, where they have been established more recently, for instance in response to workplace experience, then less time may be necessary.

Actualising tendency

A crucial feature or factor in this process of 'constructive personality change' is the presence of what Rogers termed 'the actualising tendency'; a tendency towards fuller and more complete personhood with an associated greater fulfilment of their potentialities. The role of the person-centred counsellor is to provide the facilitative climate within which this tendency can work constructively. The 'therapist trusts the actualizing tendency of the client and truly believes that the client who experiences the freedom of a fostering psychological climate will resolve his or her own problems' (Bozarth, 1998, p. 4). This is fundamental to the application of the PCA. Rogers (1986, p. 198) wrote, 'the person-centred approach is built on a basic trust in the person ... [It] depends on the actualizing tendency present in every living organism – the tendency to grow, to develop, to realize its full potential. This way of being trusts the constructive directional flow of the human being towards a more complex and complete development. It is this directional flow that we aim to release.'

However for some people, or at certain stages, rather than producing a liberating experience, there will instead be a tendency to maintain the status quo, perhaps the fear of change, the uncertainty, or the implications of change are such that the person prefers to maintain the known, the certain. In a sense, there is a liberation from the imperative to change and grow which may bring temporary – or perhaps permanent – relief for the person. The actualising tendency may work through the part of the person that needs relief from change, enhancing its presence for the period of time that the person experiences a need to maintain this. The person-centred therapist will not try to move the person from this place or state. It is to be accepted, warmly and unconditionally. And, of course, sometimes in the moment of acceptance the person is enabled to question whether that really is how they want to be.

Configuration within self

It is of value to draw attention, at this point, to the notion of 'configurations within self'. Configurations within self (Mearns and Thorne, 2000) are discrete sets of thoughts, feelings and behaviours that develop through the experience of life. They emerge in response to a range of experiences including the process of introjection and the symbolisation of experiences, as well as in response to dissonant self-experience within the person's structure of self. They can also exist in what Mearns terms as '"growthful" and "not for growth", configurations' (Mearns and Thorne, 2000, pp. 114–16), each offering a focus for the actualising tendency, the former seeking an expansion into new areas of experience with all that that brings, the latter seeking to energise the status quo and to block change because of its potential for disrupting the current order within the structure of self. The actualising tendency may not always manifest through growth or developmental change. It can also manifest through periods of stabilisation and stability, or a wanting to get away from something. The self, then, is seen as a constellation of configurations with the individual moving between them and living through them in response to experience.

Mearns and Thorne suggest that these 'parts' or 'configurations' interrelate 'like a family, with an individual variety of dynamics'. As within any 'system', change in one area will impact on the functioning of the system. He therefore comments that, 'when the interrelationship of configurations changes, it is not that we are left with something entirely new: we have the same "parts" as before, but some which may have been subservient before are stronger, others which were judged adversely are accepted, some which were in self-negating conflict have come to respect each other, and overall the parts have achieved constructive integration with the energy release which arises from such fusion' (1999, pp. 147–8). The growing acceptance of the configurations, their own fluidity and movement within the self-structure, the increased, open and more accurate communication between these parts, is, perhaps, another way of considering the integrating of the threads of experience to which Rogers refers (1967, p. 158; and *see* Appendix).

In terms of these ideas, we can anticipate clients containing, within themselves, particular configurations with which certain eating patterns or behaviours linked to appearance and weight are associated. So, a configuration may have developed that associates eating, or a lack of eating, with feeling in control in an uncertain world, or a world in which the future has been mapped out by dominating parents. Or perhaps a dominant configuration may develop that contains the many thoughts, feelings and behaviours associated with that person's eating pattern, a part of that person's structure of self that assumes a certain psychological primacy which, in turn, means the associated eating behaviours then also take a similar position in the person's life.

There may also be 'not for eating' configurations as well, or a configuration may develop or emerge into primacy that is made up of the behaviours, thoughts and feelings associated with the client establishing a different perspective towards themselves expressed through a different eating pattern. A client may also identify within themselves a configuration associated with exercise, for instance, or other behaviours that whilst linked to the eating pattern, actually have their own distinctiveness, meaning and origin. Understanding the configurational nature of ourselves enables us to understand why we are triggered into certain thoughts, feelings and behaviours, and how they group together, serving a particular experiential purpose for the person.

From this theoretical perspective we can argue that the person-centred counsellor's role is essentially facilitative. Creating the therapeutic climate of empathic understanding, unconditional positive regard and authenticity creates a relational climate which encourages the client to move into a more fluid state with more openness to their own experience and the discovery of a capacity towards a fuller actualising of their potential.

Relationship re-emphasised

In addressing these factors the therapeutic relationship is central. A therapeutic approach such as person-centred affirms that it is not what you do so much as *how you are* with your client that is therapeutically significant, and this 'how you are' has to be received by the client. Gaylin (2001, p. 103) highlights the importance of client perception. 'If clients believe that their therapist is working on their behalf – if they perceive caring and understanding – then therapy is likely to be successful. It is the condition of attachment and the perception of connection that have the power to release the faltered actualization of the self.' He goes on to stress how 'we all need to feel connected, prized – loved', describing human-beings as 'a species born into mutual interdependence', and that there 'can be no self outside the context of others. Loneliness is de-humanizing and isolation anathema to the human condition. The relationship,' he suggests 'is what psychotherapy is all about.'

'Love' is an important word though not necessarily one often used to describe therapeutic relationship. Patterson, however, gives a valuable definition of love as it applies to the person-centred therapeutic process. He writes, 'we define love as an attitude that is expressed through empathic understanding, respect and compassion, acceptance, and therapeutic genuineness, or honesty and openness towards others' (2000, p. 315). We all need love, but most of all we need it during our developmental period of life. The same author affirms that 'whilst love is important throughout life for the well-being of the individual, it is particularly important, indeed absolutely necessary, for the survival of the infant and for providing the basis for the normal psychological development of the individual' (Patterson, 2000, pp. 314–15).

In another book in this series I used the analogy of treating a wilting plant (Bryant-Jefferies, 2003, p. 12). We can spray it with some specific herbicide or pesticide to eradicate a perceived disease, and that may be enough. But perhaps the true cause of the disease is that the plant is located in harsh surroundings, perhaps too much sun and not enough water, poor soil and near other plants that it finds difficulty in surviving so close to. Maybe by offering the plant a healthier environment that will facilitate greater nourishment according to its needs, it may become the strong, healthy specimen it has the potential to become. Yes, the chemical intervention may also be helpful, but if the true causes of the diseases are environmental – essentially the plant's relationship with that which surrounds it – then it won't actually achieve sustainable growth. We may not be able to transplant it, but we can provide water, nutrients and shade from a fierce sun. Therapy, it seems to me, exists to provide this healthy environment within which the 'wilting' client can begin the process of receiving the nourishment (in the form of healthy relational experience) that can enable them, in time, to become a more fully functioning person.

Diagnosis

I have referred elsewhere (Bryant-Jefferies, 2003) to the debate as to whether diagnosis can necessarily be trusted and empirical when it comes to mental health factors, drawing attention to Bozarth (2002) who refers to his own studies of particular diagnostic concepts which do not evidence the clustering of symptoms in a meaningful way (Bozarth, 1998) and to those of others in re schizophrenia (Bentall, 1990; Slade and Cooper, 1979), depression

1990; Weiner, 1989), agoraphobia (Hallam, 1983), borderline personality-disorder (Kutchins and Kirk, 1997) and panic disorder (Hallam, 1989).

The person-centred view of diagnosis in general regards it as a language associated with a medical model of working, and not always necessarily helpful or indeed descriptive beyond the person's behaviour. This is certainly true regarding eating disorders. Yes, a particular set of symptoms may be usefully grouped under a heading but the risk is that the diagnosis assumes that the person has a set 'illness' that will be resolved by a specific 'treatment'. However, the reasons for an individual to develop problems associated with their eating patterns will be unique to them, will be the result of their own uniquely internalised meanings flowing from their own individual experiences.

Rogers also questioned the value of psychological diagnosis. He argued that it could place the client's locus of value firmly outside themselves and definitely within the diagnosing 'expert', leaving the client at risk of developing tendencies of dependence and expectation that the 'expert' will have the responsibility of improving the client's situation (Rogers, 1951, p. 223). He also formulated the following propositional statements.

- Behaviour is caused, and the psychological cause of behaviour is a certain perception or a way of perceiving.
- The client is the only one who has the potentiality of knowing fully the dynamics of his perceptions and his behaviour.
- In order for behaviour to change, a change in perception must be *experienced*. Intellectual knowledge cannot substitute for this.
- The constructive forces which bring about altered perception, reorganization of self, and relearning, reside primarily in the client, and probably cannot come from outside.
- Therapy is basically the experiencing of the inadequacies in old ways of perceiving, the experiencing of new and more accurate and adequate perceptions, and the recognition of significant relationship between perceptions.
- In a very meaningful and accurate sense, therapy *is* diagnosis, and this diagnosis is a process which goes on in the experience of the client, rather than in the intellect of the clinician (Rogers, 1951, pp. 221–3).

Vincent has drawn together some valuable passages from Rogers in relation to the question of diagnosis, emphasising that '*therapist* diagnosis, evaluation and prognosis clearly do not respect the inner resources of *clients* and their potential and capacity for self-direction, as there is an obvious implication that actually the therapist, not the client, knows best' (Vincent, 2005). He then quotes a passage from Rogers from his earlier days, yet a statement that stands the test of time, sounding with great clarity an essential person-centred perspective on this issue.

If we can provide understanding of the way the client seems to himself at this moment, he can do the rest. The therapist must lay aside his pre-occupation with diagnosis and his diagnostic shrewdness, must discard his tendency to make professional evaluations, must cease his endeavours to formulate an accurate prognosis, must give up the temptation subtly to guide the individual, and must concentrate on one purpose only; that of providing deep understanding and acceptance of his attitudes consciously held at this moment by the client as he explores step by step into the dangerous areas which he has been denying to consciousness (Rogers, 1946, p. 420).

Process of change from a person-centred perspective

Rogers was interested in understanding the process of change, what it was like, how it occurred and what experiences it brought to those involved – client and therapist. At different points he explored this. Embleton Tudor *et al.* (2004) point to a model consisting of 12 steps identified in 1942 and to his two later chapters on this topic (Rogers, 1951), and finally the seven-stage model (1958/1967). He wrote of 'initially looking for elements which would mark or characterize change itself', however, what he experienced from his enquiry and research into the process of change he summarised as: 'individuals move, I began to see, not from fixity or homeostasis through change to a new fixity, though such a process is indeed possible. But much the more significant continuum is from fixity to changingness, from rigid structure to flow, from stasis to process. I formed the tentative hypothesis that perhaps the qualities of the client's expression at any one point might indicate his position on this continuum, where he stood in the process of change' (Rogers, 1967, p. 131).

Change, then, involves a movement from fixity to greater fluidity, from, we might say, a rigid set of attitudes and behaviours to a greater openness to experience, to variety and diversity. Change might be seen as having a certain liberating quality, a freeing up of the human-being – his heart, mind, emotions – so that the person experiences themselves less of a fixed object and more of a conscious process. For the client who is seeking to resolve issues associated with problematic eating behaviours, part of this process will involve a loosening of the individual's identity that is strongly connected to the image they have of themselves linked to their eating pattern and other behaviours associated with maintaining a particular body weight or shape. It will also involve addressing the psychological experiencing that flows from their anorexic, bulimic or binge-eating experiences. Until this is 'unfixed', if you like, it would seem reasonable to conclude that sustainable change might be extremely difficult to achieve.

The list below is taken from Rogers' summary of the process, indicating the changes that people will show.

1   This process involves a loosening of feelings.
2   This process involves a change in the manner of experiencing.
3   This process involves a shift from incongruence to congruence.

4   This process involves a change in the manner in which, and the extent to which the individual is able and willing to communicate himself in a receptive climate.
5   This process involves a loosening of the cognitive maps of experience.
6   There is a change in the individual's relationship to his problem.
7   There is a change in the individual's manner of relating (Rogers, 1967, pp. 156–8).

This is a very partial overview, the chapter in which he describes the process of change has much more detail and should be read in order to gain a grasp not only of the process as a whole, but of the distinctive features of each stage, as he saw it. Embleton Tudor *et al.* summarise this process in the following, and I think helpful, terms: 'a movement from fixity to fluidity, from closed to open, from tight to loose, and from afraid to accepting' (2004, p. 47).

In Rogers' description of the process he makes the point that there were several types of process by which personality changes and that the process he described is one that is 'set in motion when the individual experiences himself as being fully received'. Does this process apply to all psychotherapies? Rogers indicated that more data were needed, adding that 'perhaps therapeutic approaches which place great stress on the cognitive and little on the emotional aspects of experience may set in motion an entirely different process of change'. In terms of whether this process of change would in general be viewed as desirable and that it would move the person in a valued direction, Rogers expressed the view that the valuing of a particular process of change was linked to social value judgements made by individuals and cultures. He pointed out that the process of change that he described could be avoided, simply by people 'reducing or avoiding those relationships in which the individual is fully received as he is'.

Rogers also took the view that change was unlikely to be rapid, making the point that many clients enter the therapeutic process at stage two, and leave at stage four, having during that period gained enough to feel satisfied. He suggested it would be 'very rare, if ever, that a client who fully exemplified stage one would move to a point where he fully exemplified stage seven', and that if this did occur 'it would involve a matter of years'. (Rogers, 1967, pp. 155–6). He wrote of how, at the outset, the threads of experience are discerned and understood separately by the client but as the process of change takes place, they move into 'the flowing peak moments of therapy in which all these threads become inseparably woven together.' He continued, 'in the new experiencing with immediacy which occurs at such moments, feeling and cognition interpenetrate, self is subjectively present in the experience, volition is simply the subjective following of a harmonious balance of organismic direction. Thus, as the process reaches this point the person becomes a unity of flow, of motion. He has changed, but what seems most significant, he has become an integrated process of changingness' (Rogers, 1967, p. 158).

It conjures up images of flowing movement, perhaps we should say purposeful flowing movement as being the essence of the human condition, a state that we each have the potential to become, or to realise. Is it something we generate or develop out of fixity, or does it exist within us all as a potential that we lose during our conditional experiencing in childhood? Are we discovering something new, or re-discovering something that was lost?

In the context of this book, we need to consider an holistic approach, with both eating/weight or size management behaviours and psychological processes inter-relating (as they do) within the therapeutic process. Each will contribute to, and inform, the other – a kind of feedback loop being generated – the system evolving and developing by feeding off the changes made and the experiences that those changes bring into awareness. The more satisfying to the person the experience of change is, the greater their motivation to pursue change further. In the context of the topic of this book, this process of psychological change, the re-balancing and integrating process then becomes evidenced through changes in eating behaviour.

Supervision

There are, of course, as many models of supervision as there are models of counselling. In this book the supervisor is seeking to apply the attitudinal qualities of the PCA.

Supervision sessions are included to offer the reader insight into the nature of therapeutic supervision in the context of the counselling profession, a method of supervising that I term 'collaborative-review'. For many trainee counsellors, the use of supervision can be something of a mystery, and it is hoped that this book will go a long way to unravelling this. In the supervision sessions I seek to demonstrate the application of the supervisory relationship. My intention is to show how supervision of the counsellor is very much a part of the process of enabling a client to work through issues that in this case relate to eating patterns and behaviours and their meaning.

Many professions do not recognise the need for some form of personal and process supervision, and often what is offered is line management. However, counsellors are required to receive regular supervision in order to explore the dynamics of the relationship with the client, the impact of the work on the counsellor and on the client, to receive support, to encourage professional development of the counsellor and to provide an opportunity for an experienced co-professional to monitor the supervisee's work in relation to ethical standards and codes of practice. The supervision sessions are included because they are an integral part of the therapeutic process. It is also hoped that they will help readers from other professions to recognise the value of some form of supportive and collaborative supervision in order to help them become more authentically present with their own clients.

Merry describes what he termed as 'collaborative inquiry' as a 'form of research or inquiry in which two people (the supervisor and the counsellor) collaborate or co-operate in an effort to understand what is going on within the counselling relationship and within the counsellor'. He emphasises how this 'moves the emphasis away from "doing things right or wrong" (which seems to be the case in some approaches to supervision) to "how is the counsellor being, and how is that way of being contributing to the development of the counselling relationship based on the core conditions"' (2002, p. 173). Elsewhere, Merry describes the relationship between person-centred supervision and congruence, indicating that 'a state of congruence ... is the necessary condition for the therapist to experience empathic understanding and unconditional positive regard' (2001, p. 183). Effective person-centred supervision provides a means through which congruence can be promoted within the therapist.

Tudor and Worrall (2004) have drawn together a number of theoretical and experiential strands from within and outside of the person-centred tradition in order to develop a theoretical position on the person-centred approach to supervision. In my view, this is a timely publication, defining the necessary factors for effective supervision within this way of working, and the respective responsibilities of both supervisor and supervisee in keeping with person-centred values and principles. They contrast person-centred working with other approaches to supervision and emphasise the importance of the therapeutic space as a place within which practitioners 'can dialogue freely between their personal philosophy and the philosophical assumptions which underlie their chosen theoretical orientation' (Tudor and Worrall, 2004, pp. 94–5). They affirm the values and attitudes of person-centred working and explore their application to the supervisory relationship.

It is the norm for all professionals working in the healthcare and social care environment in this age of regulation to be formally accredited or registered and to work to their own professional organisation's code of ethics or practice. For instance, registered counselling practitioners with the British Association for Counselling and Psychotherapy are required to have regular supervision and continuing professional development to maintain registration. Whilst professions other than counsellors will gain much from this book in their work, it is essential that they follow the standards, safeguards and ethical codes of their own professional organisation, and are appropriately trained and supervised to work with them on the issues that arise.

Dialogue format

The reader who has not read other titles in the *Living Therapy* series may find it takes a while to adjust to the dialogue format. Many of the responses offered by the counsellors, Ginny and Ian, are reflections of what their respective clients, Carol and Mandy, have said. This is not to be read as conveying a simple repetition of the clients' words. Rather, the counsellor seeks to voice empathic responses, often with a sense of 'checking out' that they are hearing accurately what the clients are saying. The client says something; the counsellor then conveys what they have heard, what they sense the client as having sought to communicate to them, sometimes with the same words, sometimes with words that include a sense of what they feel is being communicated through the client's tone of voice, facial expression, or simply the relational atmosphere of the moment. The client is then enabled to confirm that she has been heard accurately, or correct the counsellor in her perception. The client may then explore more deeply what they have been saying or move on, in either case with a sense that they have been heard and warmly accepted. To draw this to the reader's attention, I have included some of the inner thoughts and feelings that are present within the individuals who form the narrative.

The sessions are a little compressed. It is also fair to say that clients will take different periods of time before choosing to disclose particular issues, and will also take varying lengths of time in working with their own process. This book is not intended to in any way indicate the length of time that may be needed to work with the kinds of issues that are being addressed. The counsellor needs to be open and flexible to the needs of the client. For some clients, the process would take a lot longer. But there are also clients who are ready to talk about difficult experiences almost immediately – sometimes not feeling that they have much choice in the matter as their own organismic processes are already driving memories, feelings, thoughts and experiences to the surface and into daily awareness.

All characters in this book are fictitious and are not intended to bear resemblance to any particular person or persons. The fictional accounts are not trying to encompass all possible causes of problem eating, they simply highlight some of the behavioural, emotional, cognitive, psychological and social factors that can be associated for some women. Others will have developed problematic eating patterns/perspectives on their size, shape or weight for other reasons; however, the response from the PCA will be similar to that described in this book in terms of offering the therapeutic relational conditions for constructive personality change.

I am extremely encouraged by the increasing interest in the PCA, the growing amount of material being published, and the realisation that relationship is a key factor in positive therapeutic outcome. There is currently much debate about theoretical developments within the person-centred world and its application. Discussions on the theme of Rogers' therapeutic conditions presented by various key members of the person-centred community have recently been published (Bozarth and Wilkins, 2001; Haugh and Merry 2001; Wyatt, 2001; Wyatt and Sanders, 2002). Mearns and Thorne have produced a timely publication revising and developing key aspects of person-centred theory (2000). Wilkins has produced a book that addresses most effectively many of the criticisms levelled against person-centred working (2003) and Embleton Tudor *et al.* (2004) an introduction to the person-centred approach that places the theory and practice within a contemporary context. Vincent (2005) has also produced a valuable compendium of quotations and references to Rogers and his own perspectives on the theme of empathy.

Recently, Howard Kirschenbaum (Carl Rogers' biographer) published an article entitled 'The current status of Carl Rogers and the person-centred approach'. In his research for this article he noted that from 1946–86 there were 84 books, 64 chapters and 456 journal articles published on Carl Rogers and the person-centred approach. In contrast, from 1987–2004 there were 141 books, 174 book chapters and 462 journal articles published. This shows a clear trend towards more publications and presumably more readership and interest in the approach. Also he noted that there were now some 50 person-centred publications available around the world, mostly journals and there are now person-centred organisations in 18 countries and 20 organisations overall. He also drew attention to the large body of research demonstrating the effectiveness of person-centred therapy, concluding that the person-centred approach is 'alive and well' and 'appears to be experiencing something of a revival, both in professional activity and academic respectability' (Kirschenbaum, 2005).

This is a very brief introduction to PCA. The theory continues to develop as practitioners and theoreticians consider its application in various fields of therapeutic work and extend our theoretical understanding of developmental and therapeutic processes. At times it feels like it has become more than just individuals, rather it feels like a group of colleagues, based around the world, working together to penetrate deeper towards a more complete theory of the human condition, and this includes people from the many traditions and schools of thought. Person-centred or client-centred theory and practice has a key role in this process. Theories are being revisited and developed, new ideas speculated upon, new media explored for presenting the core values and philosophy of the person-centred approach. It is an exciting time.

PART I

Carol struggles with her binge-eating

CHAPTER 1

Counselling session 1: beginnings and difficulty in disclosure

Carol sat nervously in the waiting area. She knew she had 'issues'. It hadn't been easy to acknowledge what she was doing to herself, or at least not in a way that enabled her to see that she was doing herself harm. It had never felt like that and, in truth, it still didn't. She did what she did because, well, because that's what she did, and it made her feel in control. Yes, that in particular, and she liked feeling in control. It gave her lots of other feelings as well but she preferred not to think of them just at the moment.

She'd been persuaded to talk to someone about her problems. She hadn't wanted to talk to her GP, and she didn't want to see a psychologist – that made it sound even worse. And Ginny had come recommended by a friend. So Carol had agreed to make contact with her and they had spoken over the phone. Carol hadn't said a great deal, but enough to ascertain that Ginny worked with people who had 'issues', she still wasn't completely sure she wanted to think of them as 'problems' with eating.

So, she glanced at the clock, there were a couple more minutes before her appointment was due. The waiting room was in a local therapy centre, it seemed to offer a range of treatments, some of them complementary therapies. But it also offered counselling and psychotherapy. She wondered whether she might do better investing in a nice aromatherapy session, that might make her feel good. She didn't think that acupuncture was for her, though. But her friend had been quite encouraging and she had to admit that the conversation she had had with Ginny had to some degree put her at ease – well – a bit anyway. It had left her feeling heard, listened to, as though what she had said was being taken seriously. That had felt good. She wasn't sure if that was simply the 'sales pitch' and that the real therapy would be something else, although Ginny had said a little about the way she worked. Something called 'person-centred'. That sounded OK. She was a person, and she wanted to be treated as one.

Ginny had posted a leaflet to her and that seemed fairly self-explanatory. In a funny kind of way it had seemed quite gentle in the way it was written. It hadn't really read like something heavily 'psychological'. That had surprised her a little, but then, well, it had felt OK as well. Anyway, the time had almost arrived, no going back now ... She felt her heart thudding a little more, and that burning sensation she sometimes felt in her throat had returned. There was a water dispenser to her right and she decided to go over to it, try and cool her throat down a bit. It felt raw. Seemed to be worse these days.

She wandered over and took a plastic cup, holding it under the tap. It was just as she was turning the tap off that she heard her name.

'Hello, are you Carol?'

She turned and saw a tallish woman, probably late thirties, not too much make-up, brown hair, dressed in green trousers and a white blouse.

'Hello, yes, yes, I'm Carol.' She turned to greet her.

Ginny put out her hand and Carol took it. Ginny noticed that her hand was cool, maybe she been holding the water cup, she wondered.

'Hi, I'm Ginny. Good to see you. Do you want to come through, and please bring the water with you.'

'Oh, yes, yes, thanks.' Carol turned, feeling a little flustered, and took the plastic cup, following Ginny to a door on the right.

'Come on in, sit down, whichever seat takes your fancy.'

Carol went towards the seat closest to her.

'This OK?'

'Sure, whichever. There's a hook on the door if you want to hang up your jacket.'

'Thanks, but I'm OK.'

'So, I know we spoke a little on the phone and I hope you received the leaflet OK?'

'Yes, yes, I did. Thank you.' Carol nodded, and took a sip from the plastic cup, it was very refreshing, and she noticed a jug of water on the table to her right, along with a box of tissues. Hmm, she didn't feel she wanted to use those. She put down her cup on the table.

'So, you said a little, and I don't know if you want to say more, or if you have any questions or not.'

Carol was back with her thoughts before the session started. 'I liked the leaflet, it sort of made it sound easy to be here, I mean, to come here, if you know what I mean.'

'Mhmm, welcoming, do you mean?'

'Hmm, yes, yes, it sort of made it sound, well, a bit like coming along for a chat, and I know it's not that, but, welcoming, yes.'

'Like the idea of coming along for a chat is sort of more acceptable?' Ginny was aware that she wasn't really empathising directly with what was being said, rather she was responding to the sense that she felt was being communicated. It was as much about the way Carol was speaking as what she was saying.

'Well, yes, I mean, that's what Lisa, my friend, said. She recommended you. Said she knew someone who had seen you and found it really helpful – I think it may have been a relative of hers actually, anyway, she seemed quite keen. I'd sort of talked to her a bit and, well, I guess she felt maybe I needed to see someone more professional. Lisa seemed quite concerned although I'm sort of, well, I'm not sure I see it as so much of a problem.'

'Mhmm, so talking to Lisa left her feeling there was a problem, but you're not so sure, that how it is?'

'I suppose I was a bit taken aback by her reaction, I guess. I mean, I suppose I'd said things, well, we'd had a few bottles of wine one evening, bit of a girls' night actually. We go about quite a bit together, have a few laughs, you know? Had a few holidays together as well. She's a good friend. I guess it was as much because of that that I'm here. I sort of value her opinion. I mean, yes, we can really let our hair down, and have, and do, and yet there's a serious side to Lisa as well. And she was serious. And it surprised me.'

'Surprised by the seriousness of her reaction?'

Carol nodded. She didn't know whether she really wanted to say what it was. She sort of felt reluctant to. It now suddenly felt like a big step. It was like it was OK to have shared it with Lisa, that was, yes, that was OK. But now, well, she didn't know Ginny, and, well, she hadn't had a few glasses of wine. It somehow didn't feel so easy, in fact, she wasn't at all sure she wanted to talk about it.

'She's entitled to her view, but, well, it's not how I see it.'

'Mhmm, she can have her view but it's not yours.'

Carol shook her head. 'No, no it's not my view.' She felt uncomfortable, as though she was feeling a sort of pressure inside herself, and a kind of weakness as well. Her arms felt heavy and a bit 'nervy', she wasn't sure how else to think of it. She felt a bit like a child who had a secret that she wasn't really sure about and someone was wanting her to tell. And she couldn't, she didn't want to. She really didn't want to.

Ginny nodded, maintaining eye contact until Carol looked away. Ginny maintained her feeling of warmth for Carol. Clearly there was something troubling her as she was making what appeared to be a definite attempt to avoid saying much about whatever it was. Carol had said on the phone that she had a problem with eating that she wanted to talk about, but hadn't expanded on that, just that she felt she needed to talk to someone. And Ginny knew that people could change their minds, or could find that when it came to it that what they planned to say was harder to voice than they had expected. However, it was not for her to speculate. As a person-centred counsellor she saw her role as being very much one of providing a facilitative climate, offering her warm acceptance of Carol as a woman, as a person, and seeking to convey her empathic understanding of what Carol was communicating to her.

The person-centred counsellor is seeking to offer a relational climate. There is not an intention to do something with a client, or to enable or encourage a client to achieve a particular goal. There is a disciplined warm acceptance and a readiness to trust the client's process as a human-being. If the therapeutic conditions are established by the counsellor and experienced by the client then a process will occur. Where it will lead and at what speed it will proceed is unknown. The counsellor seeks to be a companion, not pushing, not seeking answers, not delving into the client's inner world, but rather openly accepting them as they are, as they need to be. The relational experience is the key to therapeutic movement.

For Carol it felt as though even in the silence that had developed, Ginny was listening, being attentive. And yet she also felt awkward and uncomfortable as well. She felt she ought to say something, but she didn't know what. It wasn't that there was pressure coming from Ginny, it was more that the pressure was coming from within herself. Say something, anything, was the urge within her, and preferably something that will take attention away from your eating.

'You must see lots of people with all kinds of problems?'

Ginny smiled, a warm and accepting smile, 'yes, I do.'

'So I guess you've heard the same things over and over.'

'Well, sometimes there may be similarities, but everyone is unique as far as I am concerned, with their own life-experience.' Ginny felt OK about going with the focus. Clearly Carol had felt a need to raise the issue and ask her question. She would have her reasons why and it wasn't for her to challenge this, but to accept it. She wanted Carol to feel accepted for who she was, for how she needed to be, and not to start giving the impression that she could say one thing and not another. All that would do would be to introduce 'conditions of worth', or exacerbate such conditioning that might already be present for Carol.

Therapeutic movement is likely to involve release from conditions of worth and from the self-concept that has been structured around them. The person-centred counsellor will want to avoid adding to the conditioning that a client may have already experienced. In order for a person to be able to acknowledge the effects of such conditioning processes from their life – often from early life which may then be built on and reinforced over the years – they need to experience themselves as being liberated from them. This may at first be slight, tentative, a kind of faint glimpse of another possibility, or a disturbing questioning that may arise towards something that had been accepted as a kind of 'given'. Only when there is a sense within the client of being 'freed up', of letting go of a fixed way of being or a way of seeing themselves, only as there comes an opening up, a sensing of other possibilities, can there be a definite opportunity for the person to question who they are, what they have experienced and how they have interpreted or made sense of the experiences.

By offering a relational experience in which the client is allowed – perhaps we might say encouraged simply by virtue of the presence of the therapeutic conditions – to be themselves without conditioning being reinforced, they may then begin to self-question. In a sense, the conditioned way of being, which is likely to include degrees of incongruence, is experienced as uncomfortable, unsatisfying, and there can then be an urge to experience something different. And, for some people, this may lead to change, and for others they may choose to return to how they were as the implications of change are felt to be too invasive, unsettling and disturbing. However, even where this is the case, arguably the client will have gained greater self-awareness through the process, an inner change that may lead to a resuming of a therapeutic process at a later date.

'But you must see some people that are the same?'

'Similarities, maybe, but never the same, not when you really listen to someone. Everyone has their own uniqueness.'

Carol wondered about her uniqueness. Wasn't something she really thought about much. She was herself, lived her life as she wanted, did what she wanted. Yes, that was pretty much how it was. Liked to feel in control, and liked to let go as well, let rip occasionally, usually when she had had too much to drink, but not always. That was her, how she liked to be. At least it was how she thought she liked to be. She did what she did and she felt OK about it. She made herself hold that thought in her mind, convincing herself that that was how it was. Yes, she thought to herself, I'm OK. And yet that look in Lisa's eyes, that expression on her face, the "you do what?" and the "oh Carol, you need some help" said in such a caring and worried way had made an impact on her. It was still vivid now, three weeks later.

Funny really, Lisa hadn't said much more about it since. But she had changed. She sort of somehow seemed more concerned, like she was sort of more serious when they were together. Yes, she'd sort of changed a little, and it had been since she'd said what she had said. It wasn't that Lisa was somehow criticising her, she didn't feel that, it was more of a consistent concern. She'd ask if she was alright. And whereas before she'd have asked it in a more relaxed and, well, lighter sort of way, something you ask someone without really thinking about it, just something you say. But now it wasn't just that. There was a seriousness now when Lisa asked her if she was OK. Yet she didn't push it. It was like she knew, and Lisa knew that she knew.

It was as if Carol had begun to feel an unease about herself that was new to her, or to be more accurate, an unease about what she did. And here she was, sitting here with a stranger. Yes, a stranger who seemed to care, who, like Lisa, wasn't pushing her in any way. Her unease was very present.

Ginny maintained her focus and her attention on Carol. As the minutes passed in silence she acknowledged to herself that silence, outer silence, did not mean inner silence. Carol looked as if she was concentrating. She looked as if "something was going on for her", and she did not want to intrude on that process. Rather, she continued to experience the warmth she felt for Carol who it seemed had something she had wanted to talk about but was now finding this difficult, or at least, seemed to be choosing not to talk about it. But that didn't mean she wasn't thinking or feeling about it. It didn't mean that it wasn't present to her now, in the room, in the relationship – simply that it remained unspoken.

Ginny did want to convey to Carol that she was present, that there was no pressure, and that it was perfectly acceptable to her for Carol to be as she needed to be. Yet she did not want to intrude or disturb Carol's silence and whatever process was occurring within her. She knew she had to trust her instincts and the urge to say something wasn't as strong as it might be. She therefore acknowledged it and waited a little longer.

Carol took a deep breath. She was aware of Ginny. Strange, she thought, sitting here. She'd come to talk and now she wasn't saying anything. Her unease had increased. She moved in the chair, feeling a little stiff. She was aware that Ginny moved a little as well. Ginny felt the urge to say something increase for her, she couldn't say why, but it somehow felt right to now say something. She trusted her experience and spoke softly.

'I feel a respect for your need for silence, Carol. I'm here if there is anything you want to say.'

Carol heard Ginny speak and looked up. She nodded slightly and tightened her lips. Her unease had grown again, but it was more than unease. Her heart was thumping a little faster. She looked at Ginny and wondered to herself. Did she want to tell her? What would happen? What *would* happen? Somehow it felt as though to say *anything* would somehow change *something*. She wasn't sure how logical she was being. She shook her head slightly, hardly aware of the movement.

Ginny had noticed the head shaking and conveyed her awareness of it. 'Leaves you shaking your head a little.' She spoke softly again, once more trying not to disturb her client's process yet wanting to convey to her that she was being attentive and listening – albeit visually – to what Carol was communicating.

The burning sensation was more present again in Carol's throat, and it was uncomfortable. She reached over for the cup of water, taking a few sips. It was cool, and it helped a little. She cleared her throat as she put the cup back down.

'There's more water in the jug if you would like it.'

'Thanks, yes, thanks.' Carol topped up her cup. 'This isn't what I expected.'

'You expected it to be different?'

'I suppose I sort of expected lots of questions. I suppose the questions would make me talk about things. But, well, this way I'm aware of not knowing what to say.' She thought as well of being aware of not knowing whether she wanted to say anything at all, but kept that thought to herself.

'Mhmm, expected lots of questions to get you talking, but find yourself unsure what to say without them.' Ginny sought to convey her empathic understanding of what it was that Carol was experiencing and communicating. She spoke with a warm acceptance in her voice.

Carol nodded as she heard Ginny replying. She was looking at Ginny again now. There was a warmth about her and yet it still felt such a big step to say anything. How would she react? Would she start telling her to do something that she didn't want to do? She didn't want that. Her throat was burning again. She reached out for the water once more and sipped it. 'I've got a sore throat, had it a while now, doesn't seem to go away.' She was looking back at Ginny again.

'I'm sorry to hear that.' Ginny was genuine in her response. She also was aware of feeling concern knowing that Carol had made reference to eating in her conversation on the telephone. She wasn't going to start jumping to conclusions, but she was aware that depending on the eating behaviour there could be throat problems, and she was thinking of people who purged themselves by making themselves vomit after eating. But Carol had made no reference to this and she wasn't going to introduce it. She kept to her empathy for what Carol was saying. 'Can't shift it?'

'No, it sort of burns, doesn't feel like a normal sore throat. I often suck sore throat sweets, they can numb it a little sometimes, but not all the time.'

'Mhmm, feels different to a normal sore throat.'

'Goes down deeper.' She felt uncertain, she knew that it often burned after . . . She put the thought aside, she didn't want to dwell on it.

'Deeper?'

Carol nodded and looked away. She felt anxious, at least she thought that was what she felt. She didn't feel comfortable looking at Ginny. Felt she couldn't look at her and keep her focus, keep herself away from saying anything . . . She took a deep breath. Somehow there was within her a wanting to say something, but she didn't want to as well. She hadn't realised she was shaking her head again.

Once again Ginny noticed Carol's head movements. She also felt that the atmosphere had changed, it felt more tense, somehow. Was it her? Was she reacting in some way to give herself that sensation? Was it something emerging within the relationship? Was it something about Carol, how she looked, her head movements, her looking away from eye contact? She didn't know, but the silence that had now begun to develop was different. It had a different feel, a different tone. Yet she didn't want to occupy herself with reflecting on her experience of the silence. She needed to keep her focus on her client. She was aware of Carol's posture as she looked down, it seemed as though she was looking at her knees. Her hands were in her lap. Every now and then they moved slightly, seemingly nervously, but she knew that could be her interpretation. Carol seemed troubled. Clearly something was on her mind. She felt she needed to communicate what she was experiencing. It felt important. She felt connected in the relationship even though not much had been said. Integrated in the relationship was the theoretical term. How Carol was being was making an impression on her, and she needed to acknowledge this.

'I'm aware of a sense of your feeling troubled by something. I don't know if that has any meaning for you, Carol.'

Carol felt herself grit her teeth. Yes, yes it did, of course it did. She took another deep breath. Her heart was thumping still faster. She knew she had to say something, but there was still a profound sense of not knowing what would happen if she did. She'd lose control. She'd give something of herself and she'd have no control over what happened next. She couldn't do that, she mustn't do that. She swallowed, her throat burned, she winced slightly. It was painful. She felt suddenly afraid, fearful and very uncertain about what to do. Part of her wanted to run out of the room, but what would that achieve? It wasn't as if she was being threatened or anything, and yet . . .

Somehow it felt as though she *was* under threat. Ginny was a counsellor, how would she react? She didn't seem to push herself at her, seemed a kind of quiet presence in many ways. That felt good. At least she was with someone who seemed relaxed, seemed warm, seemed to care in some strange way. No, not strange, but she was, a stranger, and yet she did seem to care. It made her think of Lisa again. There was something similar and yet not. She'd known Lisa for so many years now. Now, well, now they were both in their late twenties.

It is not that the counsellor is behaving in a manner to induce a sense of feeling threatened, at least she is not behaving in a threatening way, however, something within the client is feeling threatened as a result of the process and the presence of her counsellor, and how she is being towards her.

Is it the counsellor's empathy, warmth, or something about her presence as a person as she seeks to be open to her own experiencing and to maintaining her sensitivity and responsiveness? Simply by offering the core conditions a client can feel more anxious, almost as though the presence of a person who is congruent, or more congruent, has this affect on someone who is less congruent, and particularly where there is eye contact. The client is struggling with eye contact and retreating away from it.

'I don't know what to say, and what will happen.'

Ginny frowned slightly, hardly aware of her reaction. 'What will happen because of what you might say?' She sought to clarify her understanding. She wasn't sure if Carol's concern was linked to what she might say, or whether there was something else in her life that she was simply uncertain about.

'I . . . , oh, I don't know. Maybe I shouldn't have come.'

'Leaves you with a sense that you shouldn't have come here?'

'But it felt right, at least, it did when I was thinking about it before. I mean . . .' Carol took another deep breath. It was no good, her heart was racing again. She hadn't expected it to be like this at all. She had just expected a series of questions and, well, truth was she sort of half expected – maybe hoped was the reality – that Ginny would say there wasn't a problem. But it wasn't like that at all. It was much more unsettling. And she was aware that time was passing. Part of her was feeling that she could just go and not come back. Yes, yes, she could do that. But what then? What would have been the point? She wondered how Lisa would react. Lisa was a good friend. She valued that friendship. She didn't want to threaten it. She didn't think not coming to counselling would do that, but she felt sure Lisa would carry on being concerned. What then? What would she do then? She took a deep breath and looked at Ginny. She seemed very calm which was a far cry from what she, Carol, was experiencing at this moment. 'If I don't say something I'll leave here and feel that maybe I won't come back.'

Ginny nodded. The way Carol spoke, it sounded really important to her. 'It sounds important for you to say something, or you might not come back.'

'It is important. I'd sort of expected you to ask me questions and I could have decided what to say, how to answer you. But you haven't done that. You've left me to talk, and think.' She paused. 'This isn't easy and I suppose I'm anxious about how you will react.'

'Something that's really difficult to talk about and not knowing how I might react?'

Carol lifted her hand to her face and rubbed her forehead. She felt tense, felt she needed to . . . , she wasn't sure what, find some way to relieve the tension. 'I've got to say it. I'm eating and I'm vomiting. That's how it is. My friend's really concerned. I've not been concerned about it. It's what I do. It feels OK, but I'm now feeling a bit uncertain about it. I don't know. That's how it is.'

'Mhmm.' Ginny nodded, aware of feeling her own sense of how immense that must have been for Carol to say, and she felt caught between wanting to empathise with that and wanting to convey her empathic understanding of what Carol had said. 'That's how it is. And your friend is concerned, and you're a little concerned yourself now.'

Carol nodded, aware of being surprised by Ginny's response. No criticism, nothing like that. She seemed to accept what she, Carol, had said. And she seemed to somehow appreciate something of the difficulty in saying it. Somehow. She wasn't sure how. Was it her expression, her tone of voice? She didn't know. She felt heard, no, listened to, there was a difference though she wasn't sure how she would define that difference.

'I suppose I am a bit concerned. I mean, my friend's reaction, well, I was surprised. She really was concerned and she hasn't pushed it, not since I told her. And I am a bit worried, with my throat, you know?'

'Mhmm. Worried about the burning sensation?'

'It's worse after I make myself sick. Though I feel it a lot. It didn't used to be like that.'

'It's becoming more present, you mean?'

'And more intense.'

'More present and more intense.' Ginny was concerned and she knew why. Not everyone appreciated the damage that the acid from the stomach could do to the lining in the throat. And it could be serious, very serious, and now she had to make a choice. Should she voice her concern, or not?

The counsellor is aware of having knowledge that is highly relevant to the client's condition. She is unsure how much her client knows about the physiological effect on the throat of vomiting. At this point the counsellor does not know for how long her client has been purging herself in this way. To withhold knowledge from a client is arguably unethical particularly, as in this case, the dangers from regular vomiting could be life-threatening as there will be a risk of oesophageal varices; the stripping away of the lining in the throat which can then expose veins which, if they become damaged and a bleed occurs, can be fatal.

The person-centred counsellor will not want to in any way convey that they are an expert on the client's experience or situation. An important aspect of the approach lies with enabling the client to feel an expert on their own condition, life and situation. Yet here is a situation in which the client is unaware of something that has particular significance, and which the counsellor is aware of. In disclosing what they know, the counsellor is conveying an openness to their client, and an expression of genuine concern for their client's well-being. She will not be telling the client what they should, or should not do, but rather ensuring that within the client's process of deciding what to do there is an awareness of the seriousness, or at least potential seriousness, of her symptoms.

'I'm not a medical expert, Carol, but I do know that vomiting can damage the lining in the throat, and it can be quite serious.'

'How do you mean?'

'It can expose veins and lead to serious bleeding, and that's probably not something you want to hear, but it can happen. And I don't know if that is what you are experiencing, but it is what can happen.'

Carol swallowed. The truth was that she had wondered herself, but had become quite proficient at pushing the thought away. 'And vomiting makes it worse?'

Ginny nodded.

Carol felt more anxious, no, it was more than anxiety. It sounded awful. She lifted her hands to her face, covering her eyes before bringing her hands back down over her cheeks. 'What have I done to myself? I mean, it's what I do, have done for, well, some years now, on and off. I sort of go through bouts of it. I don't know why, that's how it is. I binge-eat and then vomit.' She thought to herself of her laxative use as well, but she didn't rely on that. 'It's when I binge that I vomit, though sometimes I'll do it on a smaller amount. Depends on how I'm feeling.'

'Mhmm, depends on how you feel, but it's sort of been fairly consistent over the years.'

'Started as a teenager. Kind of stopped for a while when I left home, I was 20 then. But then it started again, well, I started again a couple of years or so later. I don't know why. It was when a relationship ended, wasn't a good one and it had to end, but I'd started to make myself sick again. It wasn't a good time.'

'Uh-hu, not a good time for you?'

'I had to end it. It was out of control. It had got violent, he'd got violent. I got out. Not everyone does, do they?'

Ginny shook her head.

'It wasn't easy. I had to make myself leave, you know, I had to.' She shook her head. 'He treated me like shit but I stayed.' She felt quite emotional but was determined not to let it get the better of her. She hadn't expected to talk about this. Strange that, but she hadn't. Tommy had been a real bastard at times, and yet she still had feelings for him. It had been Lisa then who'd persuaded her to get out. She'd been right. Maybe that was why she took her seriously now.

Time had passed and the session was soon due to end. Ginny was aware that Carol was now talking about painful experiences and it felt like the session ending was going to cut across it. But she was also aware that she had to trust her client on this. And maybe it was because the session was due to end that her client had felt able to say what she had. Sometimes the end of the first session can provide a certain impetus to disclose something. She knew she could not overrun the session, she would need her break before her next client, but she wanted to acknowledge what she was hearing from Carol.

'You had to make yourself leave despite how he treated you.'

'Yeah.' Carol paused. 'Hmm. Sort of feels better for telling you that, I mean telling you about . . .' She hesitated, and swallowed, aware of the burning. 'You think I might have done real damage?'

'I'm not a doctor, Carol, but I can't deny my concern. Vomit brings stomach acid with it.'

'Alcohol can make it worse as well.'

'Yes, yes that wouldn't be unusual.'

'You think I need to get advice?'

'You feel like you want to get it checked out?'

'Not really, but then, well, I should, shouldn't I?' She thought of Lisa and knew what she would say. She tightened her lips as she thought about it. 'Maybe my doctor can give me something, she's quite good.'

'You maybe need to speak to her.' Ginny had glanced at the clock.

'I know, time's nearly up.'

'It's not been an easy session, has it?'

Carol shook her head. 'No, but I'm glad I came now even though I don't like what I now know. I do want to come back, though. I think that now I've started I need to continue. Is that OK?'

'It's fine with me if that is what you would like.'

They discussed how often to have the sessions and what was the best time and day. Carol agreed to come weekly on a Tuesday evening and the session ended.

Carol left aware that she needed to talk to Lisa about her experience and she called her when she got back home. Lisa was her usual concerned self and encouraged her to see her doctor when Carol mentioned this. And she said she'd help her in any way she could.

Ginny, meanwhile, had been left feeling quite affected by what Carol had disclosed. She wasn't shocked, but she was affected by the fact that a young woman with her life ahead of her had perhaps already done serious damage to her health. And she knew she had to accept that there had to be a reason. Yes, the violent relationship would have been a fact, but Carol had said it had started when she was a teenager. She didn't know more than that and it was pointless to speculate about it. No doubt if Carol wanted to explore this further, then she would. She rather felt that if Carol was to change her purging behaviour, well, she very likely would need to make sense of how it started, what was happening for her at the time and how it affected her. But that was for another day. Ginny wrote her notes for the session and felt her own urge to drink some cool water.

The client in this first session is quite open about her eating and this may not always be the case early on in counselling. For some clients, they will view their pattern of eating as a secret, something they do not want the outside world to be aware of.

Others will have passed through this stage and be more openly able to accept the reality of their situation and experience a stronger urge to speak about their eating and associated behaviours, even though it is likely to be painful to do so.

Points for discussion

- How would you describe Carol from what you experienced of her from this session? What feelings and thoughts has she left you with?
- Evaluate Ginny's practice as a person-centred therapist.
- How might you have responded differently to Carol, and why? Justify your responses in terms of person-centred theory.
- What were the key moments in this session?
- If you were Ginny, what might you take to supervision from this session?
- Write notes for this session.

A range of health problems can be associated with bulimia. Vomiting can cause mineral loss and electrolyte imbalance. The range of health problems include: women's periods diminishing and stopping, swelling due to fluid retention and possible kidney dysfunction. Symptoms of muscle weakness, constipation, headache together with damage to the throat, swollen salivary glands, abdominal pain, tiredness, palpitations and disturbance in heart rhythm can occur. Vomit in the mouth causes tooth enamel to dissolve. Capillaries can break behind the eyes from the strain of induced vomiting.

CHAPTER 2

Supervision session 1: reflecting on expressions of concern for a client's health and well-being

Ginny had thought about her first session with Carol, and in particular the issue about passing on information. She wanted to talk it through. She felt within herself that in her counselling role, particularly when healthcare issues came up about which she had some knowledge, that as a healthcare professional she had an ethical responsibility to convey what she knew. And she felt this quite strongly in relation to physical health issues that were quite clearly linked to a particular behaviour from a client, and where the client was unaware that what they were doing might be causing a particular problem, or were denying that knowledge to their awareness. And she also knew that another part of her questioned this view, wanting to respect the client's choices and to maintain her focus on offering and conveying empathic understanding and unconditional positive regard for her client. In relation to psychological and emotional issues, she had no problem with that. It was where there was a physical health component where she knew she was not sure.

Her supervision session with William had begun and she had been talking about her work with other clients. She now turned her attention to Carol. She described her, what she knew of her from the telephone conversation and the first session. William listened and was struck by the way that Ginny was speaking. 'You seem to have changed the way you are speaking, you sound as though, well to me at any rate, as if you are speaking more softly, maybe more reflectively, I'm not sure, but I am struck by the contrast.'

Ginny thought about it for a moment. She could see that. Yes, she could be quite animated describing her clients. But, yes, somehow she had been left maybe more thoughtful. More reflective? She thought about it. Was she?

'I think it's because I'm concerned, William, I mean really concerned about her well-being.'

'Mhmm, something she's said, something about her is affecting you in this way?'

'It's her throat problem. And the fact that she has disclosed that she is vomiting and it seems as though she has been for a while. I can just see that she may have done herself some permanent damage. And, well, I highlighted this.'

'You highlighted your concerns?'

'She disclosed how she was making herself sick – I don't know enough but, well, she doesn't look over- or underweight, maybe a little under perhaps, but it seems that she binges and then makes herself sick and she's getting an intense burning in her throat and it's worse when she's being sick and when she drinks alcohol, and, well, for me that is indicative that the lining of the throat is inflamed and maybe has been damaged. And, well, I'm not sure how much you know, but there is a real danger of oesophageal varices, exposing a vein which if it breaks can cause death. And, of course, if she's putting her finger down her throat – and I don't know if she is – to induce vomiting, that can cause damage as well.'

William nodded.

'And it's about me, my need to help her to be aware of what she is doing. I mean, she wasn't aware of what might be happening. And, of course, I know there are other problems from vomiting but it was because she was complaining about her burning throat that I addressed it.'

'Mhmm. So, you felt the need to draw attention to this medical condition?'

'I did. And I know some people might question this in terms of my being there to offer a therapeutic relationship, and not to start becoming some medical expert, but I was concerned and, well, OK, she's had the condition for a while and maybe she might have sought medical help herself at some point, but I was concerned that it might be quite bad and she might need medical attention sooner rather than later.'

William nodded, aware that he could understand the reasonableness of what Ginny was saying, and, yes, there was that issue of what her role was – purely as a therapist, or something else, something more if the occasion demanded it. 'So, you thought she needed to know what you knew?'

Ginny tightened her lips. 'Er, yes, I suppose you could say that.' Did she know what her clients needed to know? Well, no, she didn't, but was what she said likely to be helpful? She thought it could be, help her client to be more informed, or was she simply saying something to motivate her client to undertake a particular action? Or to encourage her to modify her behaviour? She knew that if she had that motivation then she was straying away from a person-centred, non-directive therapeutic focus.

'You sound hesitant?'

'It doesn't sound too comfortable, hearing it like that, but you're right to describe it that way. Did I need her to know? Well, yes, I suppose I did. But for me it comes down to my motivation.'

'Your motivation?'

'Was I trying to get her to do something or think in a particular way? Was I trying to encourage something in her, from her? That's what's important for me.'

'Mhmm, what's important for you is your motivation. Were you trying to encourage or direct something?'

Ginny took a deep breath. 'The truth is, I would like her to see her doctor. I can't deny that. The reality is that bulimia – assuming that is what it is – and I don't want to just use that label because I know that whilst it might summarise a set of behaviours and symptoms, the actual root cause can vary from person to person. So, I mean, I know that vomiting has health implications. I know it. This isn't opinion, it's fact, yes?'

'Mhmm, yes, there are known physiological effects that follow for people who vomit regularly.'

'But I only expressed concern about her throat, I guess because that was so immediate and was something that she had drawn attention to.'

'So, her physical condition was already made visible, if you like? Your intervention – if that's the right word, and maybe it isn't – but your intervention was in the context of something that had already been introduced by the client.'

'It wasn't as if I suddenly asked her whether she had problems with her throat, as one might do in a more formal assessment process. And I don't do that. I'm a therapist and I believe in working on the therapeutic relationship from the start, allowing my client to start to experience a person-centred therapeutic relationship.'

'Yes, yes, that's important. So you didn't introduce the focus from your frame of reference, but you added or should I say conveyed information to the client that she previously did not have?'

'That was my assumption that she didn't know this. Maybe she did. I didn't know. She didn't react as if it was something she knew. She actually seemed quite taken aback, and yet somehow not shocked. I don't know, maybe she was aware, well, she was aware she had a burning throat but how much concern she had, I don't know. She asked whether I thought she should see someone.'

'How did you respond?'

'She said she didn't want to see her GP, but felt she should do. I agreed with her – I can't remember exactly what I said, but I certainly wasn't discouraging her. I was, and am, concerned. I don't know that she's deliberately doing it in a self-harming kind of way, although it is in a way a kind of self-harm, and maybe if she was I'd have reacted differently.' Her comment caused Ginny to stop and reflect on what she had just said. 'Why should that make a difference?'

'If she was acting with intent to self-harm, do you mean?'

'If she was cutting herself, well, I wouldn't be suggesting she see a GP, I'd be asking her to, no, not asking her, but I'd be offering her an opportunity to talk about it, maybe make sense of it if that was what she needed to do. I'd want to understand what was happening for her, what it meant for her. I'd want to hear and to try and understand her inner world. I didn't do that with Carol.' Ginny paused again and continued to follow her train of thought. She was frowning as she sought to make sense of her sense of having made a different response.

William did not respond, aware that Ginny was thinking it through. He waited for her to continue when she was ready.

'Why?' Another pause. 'Why didn't I . . .' She stopped again. 'She was talking about how it was becoming more intense, the burning in her throat. So, OK, she's experiencing a physical symptom that seems to be getting worse. I want to try and contrast that with a deliberate act of self-harm in a more classical sense, yes? Someone who is cutting. Now, I will want to be with them to hear what they want to say about their experience, if that is what they want to do.

But suppose the cutting is getting deeper, or has begun to move closer to the wrists. What then? Would I encourage the client to see their GP? I'm sure that I wouldn't. I'd want to maintain the therapeutic contact. I'd want to be with them to help them explore what was happening for them. And yet there may well come a point at which I might say something. I mean, I could see myself expressing concern that I might be feeling.'

'OK, so, what I am hearing is that someone deliberately self-harming wouldn't cause you to respond as you did to Carol, but if that self-harming became particularly dangerous, then you might well express your concern?'

'Yes. Yes, I would. But again, yes, it would come back to motivation, wouldn't it? Would I be trying to make her stop, or to think twice by expressing my concern, or would I simply be expressing my concern because I am experiencing it, with no strings attached, as it were?'

'And that's a key point, isn't it?'

Ginny nodded. 'It is for me. What is my motivation? And it, yes, it's about my positive regard, isn't it? It's whether it is truly unconditional or not. It's about whether I want my client to behave in a different way, or whether I can accept them as they are, doing what they are doing, regardless of the risk.' She shook her head. 'And yet . . .'

'And yet?'

'I'm uneasy about withholding concern on the basis that I might be introducing some kind of conditional positive regard – a kind of "I want you to behave like this because I want you to be safe". And the reality is that I *do* want my client to be safe. What the hell am I being a counsellor for if I'm going to passively allow them to damage themselves, and perhaps unwittingly, without expressing myself?'

'Mhmm, withholding concern that is felt, experienced by you doesn't seem right to you, makes you wonder what the hell you are doing as a counsellor.'

'That's right, and yet . . . I come back to this, and yet . . . There's something key here to do with motive. It's motive that obscures something here. Let's think of me as a mirror that the client sees their reflection in. That's my role, in a sense, though perhaps not literally. But I allow or enable the client to experience themselves, see themselves. It's my job to convey my empathic understanding in a climate of warm acceptance and unconditional positive regard. That's what I seek to convey and my hope is that this is what my client receives, perceives, experiences, yes?'

'Mhmm.'

'So, the client comes to me, reflects themselves in the mirror, in this case the fact that she is vomiting and that it is causing her to have a throat problem. Fine. I can let her know that is what I am hearing and understanding. She can experience my acceptance of her as she tells me this.' She paused. 'I'm not trusting her, am I?'

'Not trusting your client?'

'I'm not feeling trust. But no, it's not that simple, no, no, it's that I'm not trusting her to do . . . , hmm, shit, that's it, I'm not trusting her to do what I think she needs to do.'

'Mhmm, so your sense of her need is not being matched by her action and so you intervene, is that what you mean?'

'Yes, because if I had stayed with her talking about how intense the discomfort was becoming in her throat, she may well have realised for herself that she needed to seek medical advice. Maybe. Maybe not. It's just that, well, I suppose I wanted to make sure, perhaps? I don't know about this. It feels like I have strayed away from my person-centred focus and yet, somewhere within all of this is a sense that there is something unethical about withholding relevant information about a medical condition given that, hmm, it's because I see myself as a health professional. And maybe not all counsellors see themselves in quite that way. I've worked in medical environments, part of multi-disciplinary teams, I am used to being in healthcare environments. I wonder. Does that leave me seeing myself and my role differently?'

'That you see yourself as a healthcare professional and this affects how you see your role?'

'I wonder. And yet . . . I keep saying that, because there is still that "and yet . . ." in relation to whether it is unethical to hold back information that I know to be factual.' She paused. 'William, what do you think? Am I losing my focus, my role, my boundary here?'

'I think that you are raising an important issue around the ethics of withholding known information. You talk in terms of a healthcare context. But how about a criminal justice context, for instance? A client telling you they drink enough in an evening to be over the limit when they drive to work the next morning. Would you convey that information if that situation arose?'

Ginny thought about it. 'I'm not sure. I don't know that it's something I know enough about to be sure of. So, I don't know, I don't suppose I would.'

'But what if you did know?'

'I don't know.'

'I do. I am familiar with alcohol units, how long it stays in the body, and I imagine I would say something. And you mention motivation. And that's important. What would it be? Well, not to show how clever I am. It would feel more about a sense of concern for my client, that they could avoid problems for themselves, and perhaps for others. There's something that feels reasonable about it, and yet, am I undermining something in the therapeutic relationship? I'm not telling my client what to do, or what not to do, but I am supplying information that might make them think and behave differently. Is that my motivation? I would have to say yes, that would be present, otherwise, why bother saying it?'

'And I think I feel similarly. To just say it without a motivation, well, why would I say it, indeed why would I be experiencing it even? I experienced concern for Carol from what she was telling me and I voiced that concern. It wasn't planned, it simply arose from being in relationship with her. She was describing her symptoms and I was able to add to her knowledge and, yes, the likelihood was that she might then act in a particular way, but not necessarily. She could have been aware of it and be denying it to herself, and could have continued in the same way.'

William smiled. 'Maybe. Maybe she has. Maybe she will. But, what you said was an expression of your concern, a heartfelt concern, a genuine experience of wanting what is best for your client.'

'Yes, but my best might not be her's.'

'So you took a risk. An informed risk.'

Ginny took a deep breath and brought her hand up to her mouth. 'I don't know. I'm not sure if there is an easy answer to any of this. I don't think there is a definite yes or no. I think there is a continuum and there is a subjective component. There is the matter of how I am touched, affected by what my client says, and that will be governed by how I am, my sensitivities, my thoughts, my knowledge, and not just what my client says but also the way that they say it. It felt right to express my concern. Yes, I introduced something, but whether it was new, or simply a development of what my client was already experiencing, is another area for debate. I expressed concern but I hope my client will feel able to make her own choice, and I hope that I will be accepting of that choice, whatever that may be. But for me, at least it is a more informed choice although, as I said before, there are other physiological effects from vomiting, damage to tooth enamel, the parotid glands can swell up, heartburn can occur and there's the imbalance of electrolytes which can have serious consequences – now I am being clever! But I wasn't speaking like that, wagging the finger, describing all the terrible things that might happen for which the client might not be experiencing any symptoms whatsoever. I stayed focused on what the client had introduced. It felt right. Some people I am sure will disagree. But, well, that's what happened.'

Person-centred counselling and psychotherapy are non-directive approaches. This means not introducing factors that are outside of the client's frame of reference. What has to be considered in this case is whether or not this has happened. Was the counsellor remaining within the client's frame of reference, merely adding more detail to what had been disclosed, or was something new being introduced?

Linked to this is the debate as to whether a counsellor, having certain knowledge that is relevant to what a client is describing, and which might reduce physiological harm if this was known to the client, is being unethical if they withhold this information. There is a professional judgement element to this.

'Mhmm.' A thought was with William that he wanted to share. 'And the thought that occurs to me is that maybe when these more advice- or information-oriented responses arise, perhaps they might be held back until the end of the session? Allowing the client's focus to flow? And then, as soon as I say that, I am aware that maybe that would then limit the time that a client might want to process their own reaction to what is being said. It's not easy, is it?'

'No, no, it isn't. But that is a good idea and somehow it hadn't occurred to me before. It had seemed only a case of whether to say something or not. And my sense that it was right to say something. But yes, the when it is then said needs to be considered and what you say, yes, I take the point about how much time the client may then have to process it, but there is a case for holding it back. And as I say that I am then wondering whether I would then lose the moment. Maybe the urge to say something is right when it arises, and maybe it varies from client to client, situation to situation. Maybe it comes back down to professional judgement on a case-by-case basis.'

As the supervision session was due to finish shortly the exploration drew to a conclusion. As can be the case, no firm decision was made as to the rights and wrongs of what had happened, but the open exploration had moved Ginny to a deeper understanding of herself and of the implications of the decision that she had taken.

Points for discussion

- What is your conclusion with regard to the issue being explored?
- Think of scenarios yourself where the matter of information being conveyed/ not conveyed to a client is an issue. If it is a continuum, where do you draw the line between what is acceptable within a person-centred framework, and what is not?
- If the client was disclosing experiences that might be considered as being psychiatric in nature, how and when might the same considerations apply?
- Write supervision notes for this session.

Counselling session 2: more history and a bad day

Carol sat down in the counselling room. She had left the counselling session the previous week aware of her need to do something about her eating pattern. Yet she also felt a reluctance to do so. It all felt so difficult. Yes, she could see that she was doing herself damage, and yes, her throat symptoms were likely to be linked to her vomiting, she understood that. She didn't like it, and she didn't really want to know about it. And yet, she didn't like the idea of having problems like that. Her binge-eating and vomiting was so much a part of her life, it made her feel secure. She had control. She liked to eat, she liked the feeling, she liked the taste, she liked the whole experience. But she also knew she did not want to put on weight. She knew that what she did made sense. She liked to eat, so she did, and to stop herself putting on weight, she vomited it back out before it could get absorbed. She didn't do it all the time. At other times she ate in a controlled manner.

At the same time, she was aware that she hadn't always felt uncomfortable about her eating binges. This feeling had emerged in recent months. Previously it was simply what she did, and it wasn't a problem because she made herself throw it up. That seemed reasonable. She was managing her binges, not like other people she saw who quite clearly just ate and put on weight, and in her view didn't take care of themselves the way that she did.

She looked across at Ginny, hoping that she would say something. She didn't know what to say herself. She'd been to the doctor who had prescribed something to ease her throat. Carol had told her what she had been doing, but that she was seeking help. Her doctor had wanted to refer her to a psychologist but Carol had said no, she felt she wanted to stay with the counselling. Somehow she realised that she was feeling good about seeing Ginny. Something about her. She seemed . . . , Carol wasn't sure how to describe it, but she just felt she didn't want to see another person.

'So, how do you want to use our time today, Carol?'

Carol thought and decided to talk about seeing her doctor. That felt easy to talk about. 'Well, I saw my doctor, and she's given me something to reduce the burning. She wanted me to see a psychologist, but I said no. She looked at the top of my throat and said it did look inflamed but she couldn't see any damage, that I should take this medicine and I'm seeing her again to see if it is helping. She's also made it clear that I have to stop making myself vomit. Trouble is, what do I do if I eat, I mean, on a binge? I haven't done since I saw her. But that was only at the end of last week. I spent a lot of time at the weekend with Lisa, and, well, I've told her what I've done and she's really encouraging and supportive. But it still leaves me feeling that . . .' She paused, unsure exactly what she was feeling other than it seemed to be a kind of anxiety and unease deep within herself, in the pit of her stomach.

'Mhmm, so you have medicine but you're concerned what will happen if you feel the urge to binge?'

Carol nodded. And she found it hard to imagine herself not carrying on as she had been.

'Just so much part of what I do, not all the time, but I just need to eat sometimes. I mean, it's a different kind of eating. That may not make any sense to you.' Carol was concerned that what she had said might make her seem stupid.

'A different kind – pattern, style, meaning?'

'When I eat, you know, I suppose normally, I don't feel this urge to keep eating. I can eat and then stop, and that's OK. But other times, I know once I start that I'm going to keep going. I just know it.'

'Mhmm, you know it.' Ginny kept her empathic response focused on what Carol had said at the end of her comments, this being the point of awareness that she had reached. She had also said it with quite a strong emphasis.

'I do, but it still happens. I mean, it's not that I've tried to stop myself, you don't think like that. I just, well, I just eat, that's how it is, and then I feel uncomfortable, and then I stop and make myself sick.' Carol knew that it just simply was what she did. It wasn't pre-planned, it wasn't something she struggled with particularly in herself although she had become more uneasy about it recently, it was simply how she was.

'Yes, you just do what you do, and what you do sometimes is to eat until you reach a point where you need to make yourself sick.' Ginny sought to respond clearly so that she could convey her understanding of what Carol was saying. She was aware of feeling warmth for Carol, and she felt sure that the way she spoke would convey that as well. She was aware that if she needed to consciously convey warmth for a client then in fact it was likely she wasn't feeling it. If she was feeling warmth, unconditional positive regard, then her words should naturally convey it.

Can a counsellor seek to 'be' expressive of unconditional positive regard? Surely the truth is that it must have a felt presence within the counsellor and then, being responsive to that experiencing, what will then be said will convey it. When a counsellor is seeking to find words to convey warmth to a client, it is likely to be an indication that the warmth is not present for them and they have an issue to explore in supervision.

Carol nodded. It felt easy hearing the way Ginny had responded to her. It felt like she understood, and that she cared. It felt as though somehow she was sharing in it in some way. It felt, yes, it felt more than anything else as if she understood not just what happened, but how it happened, and somehow that it was OK. Of course, she also felt that it wasn't OK, but she meant the OKness insofar as the fact that she did what she did. She felt accepted. She felt that what she did was accepted. Somehow that felt like a huge relief.

Ginny noted that after her response Carol had dropped her shoulders a little and had seemed to slump back in the chair.

'It's what I do, Ginny, and it's seemed OK, but now, now I don't know. And I don't know why I do it, either.'

'Now you're not sure that it's OK, and you don't really know why you do it.'

Listening to Ginny responding gave Carol time to be with her own focus. She wasn't sure that it was OK. And it felt good to have someone with her, suddenly, as she thought about it. She shook her head. She took a deep breath and sighed. 'It's not good, is it? I am damaging myself. I know that, but ...' She shook her head again. 'Where do I begin?'

'You know you're doing yourself damage, and you wonder just where to begin?'

'I don't know. It started, well, I mean it originally started when I was a teenager, like I mentioned last time, but it stopped for a while but then it started again when I was with Tommy.'

Ginny noted the way Carol was talking about "it". She also felt she wanted to clarify that what she thought Carol meant was what she was understanding.

'When you say "it", you mean both the bingeing and making yourself sick?'

Carol nodded. 'It started when I was about 15 or 16, something like that. I just sort of . . . , well, I remember I did use to eat heavily now and then – cakes, biscuits, chocolate in particular. Always liked chocolate. My parents were, well, we had what I suppose you'd call sensible food. We weren't allowed burgers and stuff like that and meal times were, well, they were sort of very, how can I put it, we'd sit down as a family. I suppose you'd say it was very traditional. And I can always remember it being like that. I mean, I suppose it's a good thing, really, but, well, it was sort of extreme. I mean, looking back, and knowing how it was with my friends. So, well, I was . . . ,' Carol paused, unsure what to say next. Meal times at home had been sort of regimented, in a way. 'My parents, me, my younger brothers, that's how it was. They were much younger than me – twins. They sort of accepted it but I suppose as I got older I didn't, but I didn't have a choice. And they were really, well, I can only say controlling about what we ate.'

'Mhmm, so regular meal times, all eating together, what you call "sensible food", and you began to find it harder to accept as you got older.'

'It wasn't just that, I mean, life at home was very controlled. That was how it was. I don't really know why, and I kind of felt that somehow there was more control directed at me rather than my brothers, but, well, maybe . . . , I don't know, that was just how it seemed.'

'So, it felt to you as though they had more freedom, do you mean?'

Carol nodded. 'They got away with things and I suppose I noticed it more after I left home. I left when I was in my late teens, flat-shared for a while before getting into a relationship with Tommy. The bingeing and being sick stopped for a while and then started again. But the twins, I don't know, things seemed to change at home after I left, things seemed more relaxed. I thought it must have been me, that they'd treated me differently. I still think that. I've said that to them but they didn't seem to want to acknowledge it. Just said they did what they did for the best.' Carol was now sitting tight-lipped, aware of feeling both pissed off with her parents and feeling that somehow maybe she had been to blame. 'Why did they treat me differently?'

'You're left with that question, "why did they treat you differently?" '

'I can only think it's because I was a girl, that's the only thing I can think of. Maybe sort of over-protective. They were like that about when I could go out, and with whom, and when I had to be back, that kind of stuff. Teenage stuff, you know?'

'A lot of control over you. Teenage stuff.'

Carol nodded. 'And I was glad to get away as soon as I could. That was a battle but, well, some friends had decided to move out and, well, we were able to rent this flat together, three of us. Good times. I really had a good time. I just went for it, I think. Lots of boyfriends, we just lived to enjoy ourselves, you know?' Carol smiled as she thought back to those times.

The counsellor has made a series of short, empathic responses, and on the last occasion her response was accompanied by a smile. Empathic

> responding has to be warm and human. In a sense the empathic responses are made in the experiential context of the presence of unconditional positive regard within the counsellor. This experience of unconditional positive regard in the counsellor in a sense sets the tone for the empathic responding.

Carol felt lighter in herself. It felt good talking this way. Yes, good to talk like this. 'In many ways I guess they were the happiest times of my life.' Ginny listened and noted that as Carol spoke it wasn't with a sense of happiness, but more with a sense of sadness. She imagined that maybe it was because it had left her thinking about how the rest of her life had felt.

'You look sad as you say that.'

'I feel sad. I mean, what were they, four years or so, I guess, then I met Tommy and, well, I don't know, that felt right, and I moved in with him but, well, he just seemed to get so jealous. I hadn't seen him like that before, it sort of grew over the months and, well, he always wanted to know where I'd been, what I'd been doing, that kind of thing. All verbal to begin with . . .' Her voice trailed off. She felt ashamed about the violence, and still felt that she was to blame, that she hadn't been right for him in some way and that it was her fault. It had been Lisa who had encouraged her to leave. They'd ended up together for a while and now Lisa was back on her own, and that felt OK, she had good friends, but the bingeing and vomiting had continued.

'Verbal to begin with . . .' Ginny noted the way Carol had looked down as her voice had trailed off, and she felt that she had withdrawn. No doubt it had brought memories, feelings, thoughts to the surface, drawing Carol into herself. Ginny felt her heart go out to her. She didn't say any more, not wanting to disturb or distract Carol from her own internal focus and process. She remained, however, focused and attentive, and waited for Carol to speak when she felt ready to do so.

Carol could hear Tommy shouting at her, could feel the fear when he had gone for her, usually slapping her on the face, but also pushing her around. Later he'd really hit her badly, and she'd end up cowering like a frightened animal in the corner of the room. He'd scream at her, accusing her of seeing other men, people she worked with, nothing more, but he didn't want to know that. He'd usually been drinking, that was when he was at his worst, you couldn't reason with him. She'd felt terrible and, well, that was when she'd started to eat, make herself feel better, sort of. It never did, and she'd make herself sick as well. Bad times, so easy to just get caught up in remembering them. They felt so close sometimes, like they were still happening. The feelings were so real, so clear, so present.

Carol nodded, thinking back to what Ginny had just said. 'Yes, to begin with. But he'd get drunk, and beat me up. Accuse me of seeing other men. Threaten me. I just wanted to hide. I tried to make things OK. I tried to be nice for him, I tried . . .' Carol lapsed into silence as she felt emotions rising up inside her, and her eyes watering.

'You tried real hard.'

Carol nodded, feeling tears break over the edges of her eyelids. 'He could be such a lovely person, sometimes, but . . .' She shook her head.

'But . . .'

Carol swallowed, it had made her throat start to burn more uncomfortably. She took a sip of water. 'I loved him . . . ,' Carol shook her head, 'and I hated him'. She lapsed momentarily into silence, 'He . . . ,' she took a deep breath, 'he destroyed me in a way.'

'Destroyed you.' Ginny kept her response flat, not questioning, simply wanting to acknowledge and not to in any way come across as pushing Carol to say more. It was a sensitive and painful time. She wanted Carol to feel in control of what she said and when and how she said it.

There are times for empathic responses to be questioning, to seek clarification, but there are other times when the client just needs to hear that they have been heard, and to be allowed to move slowly and painfully through their inner world at their own pace.

'I was really nervous and anxious. Both during and after. And, well, I'd started making myself sick again. That wasn't difficult. I felt sick a lot of the time, sick with fear. Maybe that's why I ate, to try and stop myself feeling that way, make myself feel different inside myself. Maybe. It didn't work. Nothing worked, it just got worse and, well, now I'm still doing it, even though that all happened three years ago.' She shook her head. 'Some days it doesn't seem three years ago. Sometimes it feels like yesterday. And then other days it does feel in the past. I'm still not as confident as I was. I still feel hesitant. I haven't really had a steady relationship since then. That worries me. Sometimes it feels like he just fucked me up and fucked my life up, you know?'

Ginny could only imagine beyond what she was hearing Carol say, and the way she was saying it. 'Fucked up.'

Carol nodded again. 'Bastard.'

Ginny nodded. The room felt quiet and Ginny could feel the concentration inside herself as she sat with Carol, listening to what she was saying, being present for her, with her, being open to experiencing what Carol was communicating and what was present within herself.

'A real bastard.'

Carol was still nodding. Now it stopped and she stared down at the floor, seeing and not seeing. The emotion had passed. She now felt very cold, not physically but a kind of internal coldness, a hard coldness. And an emptiness. It made her think of eating. 'Just thinking about it makes me want to eat, I mean, you know, binge on something.'

'Mhmm, the thoughts give you that feeling, that urge to eat.'

'Yeah,' she sighed. 'That's what makes it so hard. The thoughts are there, the memories are there, the feelings, they're all so . . . , I don't know, part of me. I can't ignore them, and I don't know what to do with them.'

'So much part of you . . . , what to do with them.'

Carol had begun to pick at the bottom of her sweater. Her head was bowed, she felt to Ginny even more withdrawn into herself.

Carol tightened her lips as she continued to pick at the stitches. They were a helpful distraction. Stopped her having to think. She felt herself take a deeper breath and let it out. She still said nothing, she felt no urge to speak. She continued to stare, picking at the black threads. Lost in her thoughts and yet she was not thinking. The picking was something she often did. She could lose herself. She had a sweater at home in which she had damaged the hems. It was one of the ways that she had to switch off, lose herself from herself. But she wasn't thinking about that. She was just staring down . . . , and picking.

Ginny watched, aware of feeling an urge arising within herself to want to stop Carol, wanting to reach out and communicate to her, and yet knowing that Carol was being how she needed to be. She guessed that this behaviour may occur at other times, though she wasn't certain. However, it wasn't for her to sit and speculate. She sought to maintain her heartfelt warmth for Carol, seeking to be sensitively attentive, seeking to be present with her.

Just because a counsellor feels or thinks something does not mean they have to act on, or communicate, it. And it isn't her role to lose herself in her own thoughts and speculations. Even when nothing is being said in the therapeutic relationship the person-centred counsellor has a responsibility to maintain their interior attitude of openness, sensitivity and heartfelt unconditional positive regard towards their client. After all, their role is to offer the therapeutic conditions, and that is not only when there is vocal communication. Maintaining this interior attitude is important. It generates receptivity within the counsellor and, some would argue, does affect the relational atmosphere to which clients can be extremely sensitive.

Carol felt herself take another deep breath, and she swallowed, painfully. It brought her attention away from the threads between her finger and thumb. She smoothed it back down. 'I spend a lot of time doing this.'

'A lot of time picking at the threads?'

Carol nodded. 'I lose myself. Sometimes I'm thinking, but sometimes not. I sort of go blank. Something I've learned to do.'

'You've learned to make yourself go blank.'

'Since Tommy.'

'Since Tommy.'

Carol lifted up her head. 'I can't go on like this. Somehow, I have to let go . . . I don't . . . , is that . . . ,' she held her breath before continuing, 'it's like . . . , I . . . , oh, I don't know.' She was shaking her head. 'I-I just don't know. But I can't carry on like this.' She looked at Ginny. 'It's not always like this, but some days, well, some days it is.'

'And today's one of them.'

Carol nodded. 'Today's one of them.' She lapsed back into silence, aware of feeling very unsure about herself and what she wanted to do, or needed to do. She could see that the eating pattern wasn't helpful, though it had been something that she had become used to. Except for those few years in her early 20s. 'I feel like I want to blame Tommy for it all, and yet, I mean, it was something I'd been doing before, wasn't it, though I'd stopped. I mean, I still liked sweet things, I still do, but there wasn't the intensity to it all.' She shook her head. 'I was conscious of what I looked like, though.'

'How you looked, that was important.'

'It was, well, yes, and in a way that's partly why I make myself sick. I don't want to put weight on. But it's not just that. I know it's habit as well, something I do, something, well, in a way, something I've felt sort of good about doing.'

'Feels good to make yourself sick?'

'Sort of, at least it did, but it gets wearing, you know, but somehow not at the time. I mean, it's like it's what I have to do. I eat, I feel like I'm getting too full and then I get rid of it.'

'So it gets wearing, making yourself sick, but not at the time?'

'It's like I'm in another place when I do it, and it's afterwards that I feel I suppose exhausted by it. I feel tired quite a lot. I can feel quite disgusted with myself as well. The doctor told me I'm probably undernourished, not getting all the goodness I need out of the food I eat, and other things that come up when I'm sick.' She shook her head. 'I really don't think people who haven't experienced it can understand.'

Ginny nodded, 'I can appreciate how you can feel that no one can understand, it's like it's such a specific thing that you do, for your reasons, giving you a particular experience.'

The feeling of disgust with having vomited is not unusual. The counsellor has not acknowledged this, though, in her response. We might speculate as to why. Perhaps she feels disgust herself and doesn't want to connect with her own experience. Perhaps she simply missed it and for whatever reason has felt the focus on being understood is more present.

In reading a dialogue we may not always appreciate the tone of voice, the emphasis that a client is making in what they say. Perhaps, for whatever reason, the disgust did not stand out. However, it is an important feature of Carol's experience and should be heard and acknowledged.

Carol nodded. 'Have you . . . ?'

Ginny shook her head. 'No, no, I haven't.'

'So it must be difficult for you to understand?'

'I cannot understand the actual experience that you have other than listening to how you describe it and what feelings and thoughts are present for you, and how they impact on me.'

'You try to understand though, and you listen.'

'I do try. I want to understand what it is like for you.'

'Some days I just wonder why am I doing this? And other days, it's like I accept it and just get on with my life. And then there are the days when I get that feeling and have to eat and then I'm sick and, well, then I'm sort of satisfied and then I can feel quite disgusted as well, sometimes. So many things, so many feelings. It feels too much some days.'

'Disgusted by it and sometimes it's all too much.'

Carol was nodding again. 'I can't go on like this, I know that. I mean, I think I've really begun to know that. What the doctor said and, yes, your concern, and Lisa, you've all helped me to realise that I need to change, and I think I've known it for a while but it's scary to admit to.'

'Scary to admit to other people?'

'There's that but it's most scary to admit to yourself, I mean really admit it, really accept that you're in trouble, you know? That's what's hard. Yes, there are times when I've thought I'm being silly, I should stop it, you know, but then, well, the thoughts pass and, well, that is until the next time they arise. But now, well, now it's different. I think I've known for a while, but it's taken me a while to really know it, really begin to accept it. And I think that's what's happening. And it's hard, it's so hard.' At that point Carol's emotions got the better of her and her eyes filled with tears and she broke down in sobs. 'I just want to feel in control, and I'm not. I just want a normal life. I don't want to have to think about all of this. I don't want to keep eating and making myself sick. I really don't.' The sobs continued, and Ginny sat, quietly responding to what Carol had said and to the upset that was so present.

Acknowledging the scariness has led to the client connecting with and expressing her feelings. It is important to note that for the person-centred practitioner there is no intent to promote the release of tears. If it happens, it happens. But it is not an aim. The aim is to offer the therapeutic conditions and to accept that in the experience the client will be how they need to be, and that the outcome will be a tendency towards constructive personality change.

'Yes, to be in control, to not have all of this to have to think about.'

Carol had taken a tissue and was dabbing at her face. 'What am I going to do?'

'What do you want to do, Carol?'

'Be happy. Not have to feel this need to eat, this need to make myself sick. But it's what I do. And I know I don't need to but sometimes it feels like I have to. I don't know what happens, but I can tell, I know when I'm going to binge. I feel different. I can know sometimes when I wake up. I just feel like I need something to eat, to give me ..., give me ..., I don't know what it gives me, but it makes me feel different I suppose. Because then I don't want to eat, and then I make myself sick. But it makes me feel better when I binge.' She shook her head as she felt more emotion rising and her eyes filling with tears once more, 'and yet ..., and yet it doesn't, it makes me so tired. And I ache so much sometimes as well, and the burning in my throat, why do I do it?' The tears continued, the emotions remained present. Ginny responded.

'Why do you do it?' She simply left the question that Carol was asking in the air. It had felt like she was mainly asking herself, not directly asking Ginny for a direct answer, not that Ginny could give an answer. So many things seemed to be contributing, and maybe other life experiences that Carol had not mentioned. All Ginny knew was that Carol felt the need to eat on some days to feel different, and then had to make herself sick which was in part to do with control and also to do with watching her weight. Based on what she had said. And clearly Carol now had come to hate what she did and was desperate to try and change, at least that was how Ginny was experiencing it though Carol might have a different emphasis.

'Maybe the answer has to come later. At the moment I've got to stop it. And yet, saying that, it seems back to front. Surely I need to know why, to know what I'm struggling with?'

Ginny nodded. 'As though you need to know what the cause is in order to stop it?'

'I guess they go together. I have to stop. I HAVE TO STOP.' She gritted her teeth. 'But that means not having those feelings, or not reacting to them by eating. And I need to understand those feelings, Ginny, I need to understand why I do this, now, at my age. If I were to binge tonight I need to know why.'

'Knowing why, that's become really, really important.'

Carol was nodding, feeling somewhat shaky in herself following her emotional outburst, but also feeling a certain determination.

> Perhaps the release of feelings has enabled the determination to emerge. Sometimes unexpressed emotions can be a block. Again, the person-centred counsellor does not respond to their client with the intent to unblock emotions, but accepts that this can and does occur as part of the therapeutic process and in the therapeutic climate that is being offered.

Ginny was aware that time was passing and there were only a few minutes of the session left. She drew attention to this, yet also saying that she didn't want it to cut across the process.

'I'd noticed the time a little while back. I have to make sense of it, I have to. Yes, I can blame Tommy, but so what, so it's his fault – maybe – but that isn't going to stop me eating, is it, when I feel the urge to?'

No, thought Ginny, no it probably won't. 'Thinking that way won't stop you from bingeing.'

Carol was still thinking about what she could do. She had to understand herself. She had to keep an eye on herself. She had to understand those feelings when they happened, somehow. 'What do I do? Keep a diary or something?'

'Mhmm, you could do, to ...?'

'Keep track of how I'm feeling. Would writing it down help?'

'Writing down how you are feeling when you are needing to binge?'

'Maybe. I do feel different. Maybe that would help. I don't know. But I also need to try and distract myself. I need to, I don't know, I need someone with me I think. I'll talk to Lisa. She's a good mate, she really is.'

'So, someone to talk to, be with.'

'But I have to write it down, I have to make sense of it, I really do. I don't think it'll work otherwise. I know Tommy's partly to blame, I know that, but it had happened before. He made me go back to something I did before. I say he made me. I mean, it was my way of coping, wasn't it?'

'Mhmm, it was, and it served a purpose for you.'

'It did, and it does.' She shook her head. 'But I have to find something different now, don't I?'

'Some different way.'

Carol went quiet for a few moments. 'And you know, in saying all of this, I can still feel part of me wanting to say "no, you're OK, don't change". It's there, in me. I could so easily go home now and stop off somewhere and get a large bar of chocolate – well, probably two – and eat my way through them. I mean, the really large ones. And then I'd have to be sick. Talking to you, like this, it does make me feel like that, not as much as it does sometimes, but it's there, close to me. Maybe I need to see Lisa after the sessions, to sort of help me through them.'

'Mhmm, help you through.'

'But I need to write down my feelings. I want to do that. I sort of don't want to as well, it feels like a huge thing to do.'

'Yes, you want to do it but it seems such a huge thing to do.'

The session drew to a close and Carol left feeling a range of emotions. She felt as though she had a task that she could see the sense in doing; she felt herself wanting to go and eat those chocolate bars; she felt herself wanting to just hide away in a corner somewhere and hope it would all go away; she felt good that she was seeing Ginny; she felt anxious about what would happen and whether she'd be able to control her eating; she felt tired with it all, of everything; and she was wondering how she would explain it all to Lisa. She thought about getting out her mobile phone to give her a call, then decided she'd wait until she got home. By then, though, she'd stopped off for the chocolate bars . . .

Ginny was taking a deep breath as she began to write her notes for the session. She stopped, aware that she was feeling tired herself and it seemed to be such an effort to find the right words. She was struck by the immensity of what Carol was facing up to – a habit that had taken root, and for valid, psychological reasons. And now she had to put a brake on it and make other choices. That was what she wanted, anyway. Ginny knew that Carol would do what she needed to do, but for how long would that part of her that needed control in this way, and needed her to binge-eat to feel good, last – how strong was it? And it wasn't a bad part of her, of course, just a part, doing what it needed to do as part of her structure of self. And that, of course, was so important. No good or bad parts, simply parts, each having developed for a reason, for a purpose, and each needing to feel heard and understood and warmly accepted. She wondered when she would hear from the part of Carol that was driving her need to binge-eat.

Points for discussion

- How has the session impacted on you? What are you left thinking and feeling?
- Evaluate Ginny's practice as a person-centred therapist in this session. Which of the necessary and sufficient conditions for constructive personality change can you identify as being present?
- How might you have responded differently to Carol, and why? Justify your responses in terms of person-centred theory.
- Were there any particularly significant moments in the session?
- If you were Ginny, what might you take to supervision from this session?
- Write notes for this session.

CHAPTER 3

Counselling session 3: exploring why

The session was due to begin but Carol had not arrived. Ginny was looking at the clock and wondering what may have happened. Of course, it was pointless speculating, she didn't know and all she could do was wait. She hoped that it was simply a delay and that Carol was going to attend. She was aware that Carol had given herself a goal of writing about her feelings and she wondered whether that might have made things more difficult or problematic. But then, she also knew that she trusted her to do what she needed to do and whatever had happened during the week she would continue to offer her the warm acceptance that was so important in person-centred counselling. Unconditional positive regard – she pondered on what it meant for her. Her mind drifted into the idea, presented by Bozarth (Bozarth and Wilkins, 2001, p. xii) that 'unconditional positive regard is *the* necessary and sufficient condition for constructive change as presented in Rogers' theory of therapy', and that 'genuineness and empathic understanding are viewed as two contextual attitudes for the primary condition of change; i.e. unconditional positive regard' (Bozarth, 2001, p. 173).

How did she view unconditional positive regard? It did seem important. It was different, although clearly linked to the other two attitudes. Being congruent, having an empathic understanding, feeling unconditional positive regard. That was how she differentiated them. It was as though they were each located in different areas of her experience, and yet she could see how there was something particularly significant about unconditional positive regard. It was then a feeling towards the client, perhaps more genuinely relational in some sense than the other two aspects of the therapists' way of being. And if the heart of person-centred therapy was the relational factor ... She pondered a little more on this topic.

The thought struck her that it was the therapeutic conditions that conveyed her own experience towards the client. That didn't feel quite what she meant, it was hard to conceptualise it in words, but it was something about how unconditional positive regard was in a sense her face, what she as a therapist brought, what she felt and experienced towards her client. Congruence was a state of being, how she was, and being integrated into the relationship was concerned with connection. Empathic understanding was also relational, but it was her conveying to the client what the client was conveying to her. It didn't have the same flavour of being something that emerged from herself. Unconditional positive regard was how she felt, and it was conveyed through the quality and tone of her empathic understanding and the presence of her congruence. Yes, she could see how congruence and empathic understanding did provide a context within which unconditional positive regard could manifest with greater therapeutic effect. And yet ... Somehow unconditional positive regard also seemed to be so important, setting the tone for the way or manner in which congruence and empathy was communicated.

She brought her thoughts back to Carol. Yes, she did feel unconditional positive regard for her. It wasn't something she had to make herself feel – she had reservations about that anyway. The moment you felt you had to try and feel warmth for a client was a clear indication that you weren't feeling it and immediately you had a supervision issue. If unconditional positive regard is the primary condition for change, then it had to be present, and if it wasn't, therapy was, in a sense, simply not happening.

But then, that surely goes for all the necessary and sufficient conditions? She nodded to herself, aware of how challenging it was to be a person-centred therapist. It came down to being, to how you were, what you felt, experienced, communicated, and how it was received. But it came back to the therapist's way of being. That was why person-centred working had a uniqueness to it the whole approach was centred on the how the therapist was in relation to their client rather than how they applied a range of techniques. It came back to relationship and for Ginny the notion of the person-centred approach as being fundamentally a relational therapy, or perhaps it might be thought of as 'human relationship therapy'. That certainly seemed to sum up how she felt about it.

> It is an interesting notion to think of the person-centred approach to counselling in terms of being 'human relationship therapy'. It does capture something of what is being offered. If the client can experience a healthy and wholesome relationship characterised by the core conditions, then the actualising tendency will manifest through an urge towards a more fulfilling and satisfying lifestyle which will be reflective of greater integration and accuracy (congruence) in the internal, experiential world of the client.

Ginny brought her thoughts back and looked at the clock. Another five minutes had passed. She went out to the waiting area and arrived just as Carol came in. 'Sorry, sorry I'm late. Traffic, it's madness out there.'

'That's OK, I'm glad you've made it. Come on through.'

'Thanks.' Carol followed Ginny into the counselling room and sat down. She smiled, though her lips looked a little tight to Ginny and she sensed that there was some tension.

'So, what do you want to focus on today?'

'Well, I want to go back to last week, to what happened after the session. You know I was thinking about how I felt the urge to binge. I did leave here feeling that I wanted to eat and, well, I was going to call Lisa and arrange to spend time with her, but I put it off.'

'Mhmm, so you delayed contacting her, is that what you mean?'

'I decided to wait until I got home. And then I didn't. I was already into wanting to binge. I'd stopped off on the way home and bought some chocolate. Couldn't seem to help myself. Just felt I needed it. And I got home, had a meal, but knew that it wasn't going to be enough. I had the chocolate. I also ate the rest of a cake that I had started and I just kept feeling I needed to eat something more. I sort of thought about it, but not in a way that I could really stop myself. Oh, and the ice-cream, that as well. I finished off a tub that was in the freezer. And I felt really bloated. And I drank, I had some fizzy drinks. I knew I'd make myself sick. I just knew it. And I did. And it was then that I somehow kind of came out of it and decided to write down what I felt, like we said. I mean, it wasn't really because I'd wanted to try and describe how I felt as I was feeling things, but I couldn't, didn't, I was too into the idea of bingeing, I suppose. Wasn't interested in writing anything. And even afterwards, I didn't really. I had to make myself do it.' She took a deep breath, and again sat tight-lipped.

'So, you didn't feel able to write anything whilst the process was running, but afterwards you did manage to.'

Carol nodded. 'I brought it along. Do you want to read it?'

'I'd really like to know what you experienced.' Ginny was aware that maybe Carol might find it helpful to read it, but equally she wanted to accept whatever Carol wanted.

'I'd read it but, well, it would feel strange doing that.'

'You'd feel strange reading it out?'

Carol thought about it. It would be easier if she just gave it to Ginny to read. Yes, she really didn't want to read it out. She handed the piece of paper over to Ginny, who took it.

Whilst one can debate the pros and cons of who should read something the client brings to the session, from a person-centred perspective what is most important is the client having a sense of her own autonomy in deciding this. What is best is not the issue. In reality, what is best is an unknown. How can the counsellor know what is best for the client in that moment? The person-centred counsellor trusts the client to know best what they need to do.

'OK.' Ginny felt able to accept that Carol wanted her to read it. So she put on her glasses and looked at what Carol had written.

"Another binge. Why do I do it? Don't feel too good now. Throat's burning, mouth tastes awful, feeling tired, what was the point? What has it given me? Fuck all. It's all flushed down the loo. What's it all about? I don't like myself. Feeling depressed. Hard to write much. Don't want to. Just want to go to bed, get under the duvet and go to sleep.

I knew I was going to binge. I knew it. From when I left the counselling. What's the point? What is the fucking point! Should have called Lisa, but I didn't. Think I knew I wouldn't. Said I'd call her when I got home but I knew I wouldn't, I knew it. But didn't question it. Why? What's wrong with me?

What have I done? Come home, binged, been sick, that's my evening. What's it given me? What do I feel now? I feel awful, there's nothing good. I don't feel good afterwards. Don't think I ever do. It's not about feeling good. Why didn't I call Lisa? Why? I should have. I could have. I even thought about it and still didn't. But I wanted to binge, didn't I? I wanted to binge. No, more than that, I had to. I had to. That's how it was. Had to. Couldn't stop myself. Didn't want to stop myself. Just didn't want to, now I wish I had. Now I can feel that I want to not do it, but not then. No, I'd got my bingeing head on.

Nothing more to say. Feeling like I let myself down. Let others down as well. People trying to help me. I don't deserve it. Feeling like shit. Going to bed.''

Ginny was aware of her responses to what she had been reading. She could imagine Carol sitting writing this, feeling so wretched, throat burning, unable to make any sense of it, feeling depressed and just wanting to hide under the duvet and get away from it through sleep. 'Lots of questions of yourself, and I'm just struck by a sense of how low you were feeling.'

Carol nodded. 'I binged again later in the week. Again, I knew I was going to do it. Didn't write anything, didn't see any point. Wasn't anything different, maybe more frustrated with myself. I just don't see what I get out of it. It's hard to think about what I'm doing when I'm eating like that. I don't think the same as I usually do. I mean, I just seem to go for it, I just do it. My head changes. I don't know how else to describe it.'

Ginny stayed with the language that Carol was using. 'It feels like your head changes? I'm not sure I understand exactly what you mean by that.'

To just reflect back what the client has said does not necessarily convey to the client any sense of the counsellor understanding what they are seeking to convey, and what they are experiencing. At best it may tell them that the counsellor is listening, and maybe sometimes that is all the client wants, to feel listened to. But there are times when the client wants, needs, more than that. They want to feel heard *and* understood. Here, the counsellor hears the words but is unclear what they mean. So she asks. This is good. It conveys to the client that the counsellor wants to know, that it matters to them to know. Obviously, tone of voice will also be important to ensure that interest is conveyed.

However, this is not a case of probing the client for answers and more detail. There is no intention to put the client on the spot. That would not be person-centred. This is about the counsellor clarifying her understanding so she can be sure that she has heard and understood what the client is experiencing and seeking to convey.

'It's like I'm somewhere else. Like being out of it, but I'm not. I mean, sort of like being a bit pissed, but it isn't.'

'Somewhere else, out of it, bit like being pissed but . . .' Ginny moved her head from side to side, '. . . but not exactly?'

'No, I mean, I don't know, it's really hard to describe. I just get it in my head and that's it.'

'Mhmm, you get it in your head to binge and that's it, it feels sort of inevitable.'

'It feels like I don't have any choice. I have to. And I really mean that. I HAVE to.'

'Mhmm, no choice, you just have to do it, not even a sense of having a choice.'

'No, no. I mean . . .' Carol thought about it. 'I suppose I do have a choice, but I don't. It doesn't feel like I have a choice. I'm not thinking about choosing something else. I mean, after I left here, yes, I thought about phoning Lisa, I could have done, but I didn't. I thought I'd call her from home. I sort of convinced myself that this was OK, but I didn't really need to convince myself. It wasn't that I needed convincing, I just decided that was what I would do, but I think I knew that I wasn't going to. And, yeah, and I wasn't sort of worried about that. Like I say, I'd already got my bingeing head on – that's what I call it.'

'So, your bingeing head is on and that's it, you're going to binge, nothing's going to get in the way of it happening, and you're not even thinking about it as a choice, it's what you're going to do, didn't worry you.' Ginny really felt it was important to try and communicate as fully as possible what she was experiencing from what Carol was saying. She wanted Carol to feel heard and understood. She was also aware of feeling acceptant of what Carol was saying. She had no feelings of criticism, no sense that Carol should have had more control, or anything like that. No, she felt warmly accepting of Carol and of her experience. And she wanted to understand, to be clear as to what Carol had experienced and was experiencing.

'No, not at the time. Afterwards, yeah, when I tried to think about it. But it's too late then, isn't it?' Carol paused shaking her head. 'Why do I do it? I have to understand it. I have to know what it is that happens. It's like it's me but it isn't me. I mean, it is me, and, well, I guess it's part of who I am. It's what I do.' She shook her head again. 'But why? I mean, OK, yeah, I know about Tommy and that and, well, yes, but he's not around any more, thank God.' And as she said that she also felt a pang of loss as well. She hadn't really ever got over him. Such a bastard to her and yet she knew as well how he could be. But he'd get drunk, get jealous and she knew she couldn't cope with that again. What a couple. He'd lose it and get violent and abusive, she'd lose it and eat. Was that how it was?

'No, he's not around. But it feels like it's part of you, though it sort of isn't you?'

Carol thought about it some more. 'I don't know. I want to know but then, well, sometimes I don't want to think about it. I just want it to all go away.' She stopped again. 'You know, I'd be OK if I could just binge when I wanted and, well, didn't have to worry about the effect it was having on me. And sometimes, I mean, I don't always think about that either.'

'Don't always think about the effect it has on you?'

Carol shook her head. 'Don't want to know . . . but I do as well. Oh I don't know, I get confused by it all, I just want to feel OK, that's all. Is that too much to ask?'

'Just want to feel OK, that's really important. Feels like it isn't too much to ask.' Ginny emphasised the importance because of the way Carol's voice had increased in volume and pitch.

'When I didn't think it was a problem it was easier. Now I know it's a problem – though not when I've got my bingeing head on – then it's not a problem. Then nothing's a problem.'

Ginny nodded. 'Like it's worse now because some of the time, when you're not bingeing, you know it's a problem.'

Carol was thinking about what she had said as Ginny was responding. Her thoughts had gone back to her bingeing experiences. 'I just need to eat. Usually sweet things, but I can go for crisps as well, and those little cheesy biscuits, and corn chips, that kind of thing. But chocolate, ice-cream, cakes, cheesecake as well, that's what I go for.' She shook her head. 'And what do I get out if it? What do I really get? Does it make me feel good? No. And yet, and yet it sort of does, it must do. I mean, oh I don't know, it's really hard to talk about it.'

'Feels hard to talk about.'

'I feel ashamed about it, I feel as though I ought to be able to be different.'

Ginny noted the shift from talking about to expressing what was present for her in the here and now. 'You're feeling ashamed, feeling you ought to be different.'

'Feel like I don't deserve any help.'

'Mhmm, like you don't deserve having anyone helping you.'

Carol was looking down and shaking her head. 'Don't deserve it. I'm crap, what's the point.'

'Feel like crap, no point in being helped.'

The counselling interaction has brought Carol to a place in herself where she engages with feelings about herself that underly her attitude to being helped and helping herself. Again, it has not been the counsellor's intention to reach this place, but it has naturally happened as a result of the offering of the therapeutic conditions. The person-centred counsellor trusts this as being a necessary part of the client's process. Now the client needs to feel warmly supported and accepted in her experience towards herself.

The room felt quite silent. It felt important to Ginny to stay very alert and attentive. It felt as though Carol was becoming her feelings in a more present and immediate way in the session and in the relationship. She didn't want to say or do anything that might disturb that focus, that process of becoming what she was feeling. However, her heartfelt warmth for Carol remained very present, and she felt good about feeling this way. It was important to her to naturally be in touch with that response.

Carol felt suddenly very small, weak and helpless. It was not an unfamiliar experience and was something she rarely spoke about. It brought with it memories, vivid memories, of hiding, trying to protect herself from the verbal and physical onslaught. It would leave her feeling dead inside, and that was how she felt now. She didn't speak. She had no words to say, there were no words, it was just too sickening to begin to try and describe.

For Ginny it felt as though Carol had retreated away from her and into the chair. The silence seemed more intense and she held her focus, aware that she had begun to frown, a sign of her concentration. She relaxed her forehead and waited. Her feelings of unconditional positive regard for Carol remained very present.

Carol could feel her body wanting to shake, it began haphazardly – she was used to this happening from time to time. Her muscles would twitch and she would just move in a way she could not control, and then it could spread so that she just felt herself shaking. This was what was happening now. It made her breathing very disjointed. She felt light-headed, and sick, sick in the very pit of her stomach, but not normal sickness, this was a sickness rooted in fear. Only Lisa had seen her like this – and her doctor who had given her some pills to try and relax her. But she'd only prescribed them for a while, saying they could be addictive and she didn't want Carol to have that kind of problem. They had helped, at the time it had been really bad, just before she had left Tommy. Nowadays, if it happened at home, she'd have a drink, that would calm her down. But she controlled it. She was wary of using alcohol too much like that.

'Sorry, but I get like this sometimes.' Carol spoke through the shaking that was continuing.

'Happens when you feel like this?'

Carol nodded, and took a deep breath and held it, trying to control the shaking. 'I think about things, things that have happened to me, Tommy,' she sniffed, 'being beaten and slapped about.' She swallowed and sniffed again, feeling the tears building up in her eyes. The shaking dislodged them and they ran down her cheeks. 'Made me feel like I was just shit, nothing, no one,' another deep breath which she held again. The shaking continued. The sickly fear remained deep inside her. 'Fucking bastard.' Her breathing remained very jerky. She closed her eyes, more tears flowed. Another deep breath and she swallowed again before breathing out. The next deep breath and she tried to get some control. She swallowed again. 'Fucked me up, Ginny, he fucked me up.'

'What he did, yeah, makes you feel so fucked up.'

Carol nodded, her head movements were still very jerky. Yeah, she thought, fucked up.

Ginny was aware of not knowing exactly what Carol meant by "fucked up", but she set it aside. She needed to remain with Carol in her experience. Her warmth remained very present, her heart went out to her. And she noted feelings of anger towards this Tommy as well. She took a deep breath herself, but quietly, not wanting to distract Carol from her focus.

Carol was taking another deep breath herself, 'I just feel like . . . , what's the point. What's the point in living? And that's stupid, I know that. But there have been times in the past when I've wanted to, you know, thought I'd be better off dead.' She closed her eyes as she felt another surge of shaking coming on. 'I-I ne-ne-ne-ver d-did an-an-any-thing. I couldn't. But I thought about it.'

'You felt like it, thought about it, that you'd be better off dead, though you never did anything.'

Carol shook her head. The latest waves of shakes were easing. 'I just feel this awfulness inside me, cold and . . . , it's like your insides are sort of, . . . , I don't know how to describe it, like it's sort of churning but it's kind of deeper than that, and it's cold, and it's numb. Numb.' Carol shook her head. 'How can it be numb when there's this awful feeling as well?'

'Churning, cold, and awful feelings, and numb, as well.' Ginny wanted to convey what she understood Carol as saying. She didn't voice it as a question as this would have directed Carol to explore the contrast between the numbness and the awfulness. If she wanted to do that then she wanted to leave Carol free to do this by her own choice. She simply wanted Carol to know what she had heard.

> The counsellor's responding does not disturb the client's affective focus. She is being what she feels.

Carol suddenly shuddered. She still had her eyes closed. 'It's like my arms, I feel it in my arms, they go numb, heavy, like they're sort of not mine, sort of. But inside me, it's fear, no it's more than fear, terror. Utter terror. I never know when it's going to be there. Makes it hard to go out, sometimes, makes me want to just hide away for the day. Sometimes I do, go sick, but other days I make myself go into work.' The shaking had subsided and it had left Carol feeling drained and sort of distant from herself, like she was slightly separated off from herself, from her feelings. 'There's that numbness now, like I'm sort of not feeling.' She shook her head. 'I know they're there but I'm not feeling them.' She thought for a moment, she was making a connection that she hadn't really thought about before. 'Hmm, bingeing does that. Bingeing stops me feeling, hmm, makes me feel, well, different. Uncomfortable! Is that why I do it? No, that can't be right. I was bingeing well before I met Tommy.' She looked up towards Ginny.

'Feels like you binge to go numb, is that what you mean?'

> The focus has shifted from the feeling and into thinking. This is the client's process, the counsellor has followed it.

'I'm not sure. Maybe it is, at least, it is with these feelings, but that wasn't why I binged in the past.' She stopped again and frowned. 'I mean, in the past it was sort of, well, being able to do what I wanted, having control over myself. Eat the things I never did, but then I'd make myself sick because I didn't want to put on weight. Thought I'd got it sussed, you know?'

'Mhmm, seemed like you had it sussed, eat to experience what you didn't have before, and make yourself sick to not put on weight.'

'Makes sense, doesn't it? It did. It still does. But that was then. That was different.' She paused as she sought to grasp what she was saying. It seemed important, somehow. What was it? 'That was different.'

'Different?'

'In the past, I mean, I binged and made myself sick, and that was about being at home, having some control. I can see that. Then I was doing it because I was having what I wanted, but going over-the-top. That was like different. Hard to describe it though.'

'Let me see if I am understanding you. Bingeing at home, at the start, that was to do with control.'

Carol nodded, 'feeling in control. I'd eat, and then I'd make myself sick. Not all the time, but a lot of the time. As I got older I made my own choices and, well, then I was having to make myself sick to stop weight gain. I was quite slim – still am though not like I was then. I could be like the girls in the magazines. So, being sick just helped with that. I had control. I could make myself be as I wanted to be.'

Ginny nodded, 'you found a way to be how you wanted to be. You had control.'

'But I didn't set out to do that. I don't think. It was control, my control. I had to eat, it was that kind of family, so I couldn't be, you know, like an anorexic and starve myself. You ate, that was how it was. So I took control by throwing it back up. And then I realise that actually that helped, helped to make me look how I wanted to look.' She shook her head. 'I suppose these are things that I've known but haven't really talked about much. I mean, I sort of knew them but didn't. I mean, it doesn't make sense as to why I do it now. I'm not thinking like that. I don't understand why, like last week, I had to do it? That doesn't make sense. I'm able to choose what I eat. I have the control I didn't have at home. So why do I still do it? So it comes back to Tommy and how he made me feel, doesn't it?'

'It feels complex listening to you, with different meanings for your bingeing and being sick at different times of your life, yes?'

Carol nodded. 'Like it's the same behaviour, but for different reasons at different times, and yet . . . ,' Carol could see that there was a link, nevertheless, '. . . and yet, there is a link, and that's control.' She paused again. 'But what do I need control over now? I don't understand that.'

'What do you need to control now, you mean?'

'I don't, well, except for when I feel like I have today. But I don't always feel like that, I didn't last week, I don't remember feeling like this and then deciding to binge – not that I felt like I decided to, I just did it.'

'Just did it, no control.'

'No control and yet feeling I'm in control.' She shook her head. 'It all seems so confusing.'

'Confusing to feel in control and not in control.'

'The only thing I can't control at the moment is what is happening inside me. Work is OK. Social life is OK. But not what I feel about myself sometimes.'

'You can't seem to control how you feel about yourself, some of the time.'

Carol nodded. 'And I can feel pretty low, you know, and I can lose myself in my memories. And I don't want that, but it happens. But I don't sort of decide to go and binge, in fact, thinking about it, when I feel really bad like that I just want to go to bed, go to sleep, hide. I mean, sometimes I'll eat, but when it's really bad I don't think I do.'

'So when it's really bad, you don't think you binge, but when it's sort of less than bad – if that's OK to put it like that – then you may binge?'

'It's like there are different levels to it.'

'Different levels to what you feel?'

Carol nodded, suddenly feeling good, as if she had got hold of something that sort of made sense, seemed to help her to feel more able to understand herself.

'Yes, different levels. Like I can feel so bad that I don't want to do anything. That's when it's really deep, I mean, you know, that fear, terror, it's in me, I can feel it'. She put her hand over the pit of her stomach. 'I just can't do much when I'm like that. But that's not so frequent as it was. I mean, with Tommy it was sort of always there, particularly in the evening waiting for him to come home, not knowing how he would be. And yet, I did eat, then, and I drank. Enough to calm myself. Still do sometimes to calm myself, but not like I did. I've controlled that.' She had never really liked alcohol. Much preferred the effects of eating. But she did drink, and had had bouts where it had been important. But she'd had to control it as if she'd been drinking too much that could set Tommy off as well. She'd just had to be so careful.

'I spent my life walking on eggshells, never knowing what might cause a problem, and sometimes I did nothing, and that was when it was worse, I didn't know what I'd done. I didn't know. But there wasn't anything, it was him, but he made me doubt myself, made me feel that it was all my fault. That's what made it hard for me to leave. I thought it was my fault. It's crazy, looking back, and yet that's what he did to me. I've had to get over that. And I can still doubt myself, I still get anxious, not sure if I can do something new that I'm, say, asked to do at work.' She shook her head. 'I'm not sure I'll ever really get over that.'

'Feels like that self-doubt has taken root inside you.' Ginny used her own imagery. It was expressive of the sense that she had as she listened to Carol speak.

'I'm not as confident as I could be, should be. When I'm out, a couple of drinks loosens me up. Then I'm fine.'

'A couple of drinks loosens you up, makes you feel more confident.'

Carol took a deep breath and breathed out slowly. 'What a mess, huh?'

'Feels like a mess?'

'Feels like wreckage, I mean, it feels like . . . , yes, I don't know why that idea came to me, but I can't think of any other way of saying it, it does feel like wreckage, after a sort of storm has not exactly destroyed everything, but it's like it's blown the windows in, thrown everything around inside.'

'And that's how you feel, like your windows have been blown in, that you've been thrown around inside?'

Carol nodded, taking another deep breath as she did so. 'Windows punched in would be more accurate.'

'Windows punched in.' She paused momentarily, 'Tommy.'

Carol nodded again.

'Tommy.' Carol was shaking her head. 'I can see that. And you know it's like I've boarded myself up. That's what I sort of do when I go to bed, sort of board myself up, stop him, it, getting to me.'

'You board yourself up to stop him, it, getting to you.'

'But I'm amongst the wreckage, I am the wreckage, that's how I feel sometimes. I am the wreckage.'

'You are the wreckage.' Ginny spoke softly as she felt Carol's own tone of voice convey a sense of increasing self-reflection.

'And somewhere in all of this I got bulimic.'

Ginny noted that this was the first time that Carol had used that word to describe herself. For whatever reason, it was now feeling OK for her to say it – not that she knew whether or not it had felt OK before – but it was a word that she was now using, and it felt important that she convey that she had heard this.

Not all clients will want to use the language of diagnosis. Yet for some people it will be something they want to do to be able to define what they are experiencing. It is an individual choice. Whether or not a client wishes to use a particular term to describe what they are experiencing or how they are behaving is up to them. Does it have meaning to them? Does it help them define who they are, in some way? Is it a definition that they want? And, of course, however dominant the symptoms may become, people are more than their diagnosis, even if that 'more than' is held as potential rather than in evidence at the time.

'Somewhere in amongst the wreckage you got bulimic.'

'And like we were saying before, different levels, different times, different reasons, maybe. It's not just simply being bulimic, is it? There's all these reasons why. I've never thought like this before, not really, not like we've talked today. And it's nearly time to finish.'

'It's felt very important, and I do hear you say that it's new to you to think like this.'

'I can sort of see it more clearly. I started making myself sick to have control at home, then to control my figure, then as I binged more to eat what I hadn't been allowed before I had to be sick more to keep my figure. Then I was away from home, living with friends, and it all settled down. Then Tommy, and he made me feel so awful and I went back to eating, I suppose to feel in control of something, though I wasn't really in control of anything. And I still do it, but now, well, what I need to feel in control of is me, what's happening inside me.'

'That sounds really profound, Carol, like you've found a way to sum it up so clearly, and now it's about feeling in control of what's inside you.'

'The wreckage. It's like I've got to put myself back together. Like I've been, I don't know, sort of taken apart. And you know, can you do that? I mean, imagine you make a cake and you use the wrong ingredients, or the wrong quantities, and you cook it at too high a heat, say, or for too long, and you get, well, you get what you get, but it's no good. The ingredients are in it, but it's not very nice. I mean, you can't take it apart, can you? You'll just have a plate of crumbs, and burnt crumbs at that.'

'That how it feels?'

'Sort of. But then, I also want to say that maybe it's only part of the cake that's messed up. That sort of doesn't make much sense talking about a cake. But if you could have a cake that's OK in part and then another part's messed up with the wrong ingredients and is over-cooked. And some of them get into the good part as well. What do you do? You can't take it to pieces. What do you do?'

'You don't feel you can take out of yourself the bits that are messed up?'

'Cake's not a good analogy. Maybe a plant that's died, or at least, some of it that has.'

'OK, so, what would you do with that?'

'Cut out the dead stuff and encourage it to grow.'

'Mhmm.' Ginny didn't say any more, she wanted to let Carol remain with what she had said for within that there was a way forward – though Carol would have to translate it into her own life with her own meanings.'

'Hmm, easy to say, cut out my dead wood. But you know more important is to nurture the new, is that what you mean?'

Ginny was aware of not having said anything. 'Is that what it feels like to you?'

'And I guess that's what I need, to feel nurtured.' She paused. 'That's what this is about, isn't it?'

Ginny nodded.

'And I need to make other choices and changes to help with this, don't I?'

'Probably.'

'Hmm. I have a lot to go away and think about, a lot. This hasn't been easy, but it has been so helpful.'

The session drew to a close and Ginny sat back in the chair after Carol had left, to reflect on what had been an incredibly intense and yet such a rewarding session. It had been as though Carol was suddenly ready to start to make connections, even after that difficult emotional release earlier in the session. Clearly Carol had the capacity to self-reflect and she knew that not all her clients were so proficient in this. She knew she was interested in hearing what Carol was going to do with her insight, how it was going to affect her.

So many contradictions, which Ginny knew seemed to be a feature of any kind of addictive behaviour. Her eating pattern in a sense was out of control, and yet actually very controlled. There were so many reasons for it developing into bulimia, each playing a part, each contributing a particular meaning to the act of bingeing and of vomiting back out. And Carol was now calling it bulimia as well. That was interesting. But at least she had come to the point of using this term after acknowledging the complexity. She felt sure that Carol was seeing bulimia as a behavioural effect, rather than as a classical "disease" that you catch, a behavioural effect of a way of experiencing herself in relationship with others, expectations of society and with herself. Fucked up, messed up, punched in, wreckage – powerful words conveying powerful images. She could see that a lot of sifting through the wreckage might be needed, to be able to be sure what is "dead wood" and what is able to come into bud, as it were. Messy mixing metaphors like this, but life was messy. People were complex, and difficult experiences seemed to enhance the complexity of it all.

Carol called Lisa straight after the session. She was not going to risk anything happening like the previous week, she'd already talked to her about this and they'd agreed to meet up. Carol just needed to check that Lisa wasn't delayed. Actually, Carol felt different this week, not the same urge to eat. She was somehow more "in her head" and it wasn't her "bingeing head" either. So much to think about, so much to sort out in herself. It could have felt all too much, but somehow it didn't. She felt a certain enthusiasm. Why had she started talking about a cake? She was shaking her head to herself. And yet it did feel like that. A real mess of ingredients. And yet, she felt sure it wasn't completely messed up. Yes, there were days when she felt like she was, the really bad days, but they didn't happen so much, it was more this sudden urge to binge that got hold of her. She knew she had to make changes in her life, get some more things in to nourish her. She liked that idea. Maybe she needed a holiday, sun, somewhere quiet. A Greek island maybe, but a quiet one. That was different. Usually she'd have been thinking of somewhere much more alive, but that somehow didn't appeal. She wondered if Lisa would be up for it? It would be different. Maybe it was what she needed right now.

Points for discussion

- What thoughts and feelings are most present for you, and why? What are you left thinking and feeling?
- How do you react to the complexities indicated as lying behind bulimic behaviour?
- Evaluate Ginny's practice as a person-centred therapist in this session.
- How might you have responded differently to Carol, and why? Justify your responses in terms of person-centred theory.
- What were the significant moments in the session and what contributed to their occurrence?
- If you were Ginny, what might you take to supervision from this session?
- Write notes for this session.

CHAPTER 4

Counselling session 4: feeling low, everything's a struggle, need to get a life

'I'm making changes, but I'm having really low days as well. It's like I'm feeling better, and I'm feeling worse.' Carol sat in the chair in the counselling room, feeling somewhat bewildered by it all. She'd left the last session on something of a high, feeling positive, but it had been anything but a smooth week. She'd spent a lot of time with Lisa. She'd managed not to binge, but it had been hard, so very hard. She knew she'd used Lisa's company a lot to distract herself, but she also wondered if that was really what she should be doing. Lisa, though, seemed OK with it. But she didn't want to put strain on their relationship. Lisa was so supportive.

Lisa had really listened as well to what she had been saying after the last session. Going over it again made it seem to make more sense. And feeling positive had lasted a couple of days, and then she'd felt low, but had managed to get into work and it had eased. Then it had sort of felt OK, and then at the weekend she had gone down, had a really bad day on Saturday. Lisa had been around and they'd talked. It hadn't been easy to talk to her, but she had managed to, and it had eased and by Sunday she was feeling her spirits lift a little. Sunday had been a sunny day as well, not that Saturday had been bad, but she hadn't taken much interest in it. She didn't when she felt like that. Nothing seemed to hold much interest.

'Better and worse, up and down? Can't be easy.' Ginny had noted the confused look on Carol's face as she had been speaking.

'No, but, I guess that's what happens. Lisa's been great, and I learned so much last week, so much began to make sense.'

'Mhmm. You could begin to start making sense of what you experience?'

Carol nodded. 'I really crave eating some evenings, well, most evenings. It's just there, and it's hard to distract myself when I'm on my own. I just don't feel right. Feel anxious, just can't settle down. And then I don't sleep well, and that makes it worse. I'm tired and it's so easy to give up. And I know I don't want that as well. But, at the moment, it's really hard.'

Ginny could see from the expression of Carol's face that she was having a hard time. 'I can see the struggle in your face, Carol, wanting to not binge and yet feeling that craving in the evenings.' She spoke with warmth, acknowledging the struggle that Carol was having with herself.

Empathy is not only about responding to words. The facial expression of the counsellor in response to the client's expression is important. And, further to this, is the expression in the counsellor's eyes. Where there is a heartfelt experience of unconditional positive regard towards the client then warmth will be present in the eyes. The presence of eye contact, and the nature of eye contact, are highly significant factors in the therapeutic process and can offer opportunity for a lot of unspoken communication of the therapeutic conditions.

Carol felt good that Ginny cared. She could feel that caring, hear it in her voice, see it in her eyes. That meant a lot to her, but it didn't help her when she was sitting at home desperate to binge on something, anything which she knew that inevitably she would then have to make herself sick to get rid of. And she didn't want that either. Here she was trying to control her eating, and she felt more out of control than ever. She knew she couldn't binge, she didn't want to put on weight, and if she did, well, she could only do what she always did. And she couldn't, she felt torn apart, and knowing how much she was currently feeling very dependent on Lisa, and that wasn't fair on her.

She didn't feel like saying anything. It had been a struggle to get to the session. Now she was here she just wanted to ..., she wasn't sure, just sit, or go home again? No, she didn't want to go home. She'd eat, she felt sure she would. And she'd feel bad about leaving. That wasn't an option. She'd stay, maybe she might start to feel different, but she wasn't feeling too optimistic. And she was so tired as well, not sleeping so well was really taking it out of her. She yawned. 'Sorry.'

'You're tired.'

Carol nodded. She didn't say anything. She didn't feel like saying anything. It just felt suddenly like all too much effort. Everything felt like too much effort. What was the point. Was every day going to be like this? Was this going to be her future, always struggling with herself? She didn't even feel she had the energy to try and think about it. It was all too much.

Ginny meanwhile had noted how Carol's body language seemed to be suggestive that she wasn't just tired, but that she was struggling to make an effort. She seemed slumped in the chair, staring slightly down, and it was a kind of stare. She seemed lost in thought. She wanted to communicate her sense of how difficult it seemed for Carol at the moment, but simply so as not to disturb or distract her too much. 'Tough place to be.'

Carol heard Ginny and felt herself nodding slightly. She was also aware of feeling afraid as well, afraid of not being able to control her eating and vomiting, afraid that her bulimia would get back in control – control again. Either it's in control or I am ... But she didn't take her thoughts any further, she simply didn't have the energy. She continued to sit in silence, staring blankly, lost in her inner world which, at that moment, was feeling quite empty.

Ginny stayed with the silence, maintaining her feelings of warmth and her attitude of unconditional positive regard. She accepted Carol's need to be as she was, silent, saying nothing, staring in a manner that seemed quite blank. It was, she imagined, expressive of what she was experiencing inside herself. Today, now, this was what was present for – or should she say within – Carol. Maybe she had struggled to a kind of standstill. For Ginny, there was a core acceptance of her own need to maintain the therapeutic conditions, be open to her own experiencing whilst holding her feelings for her client, and being ready to respond to express empathic understanding of anything that Carol might wish to communicate. At the moment she was communicating silence. Ginny conveyed her empathy by respecting this, and being silent herself.

It was strange, Carol was aware of sitting, and of thinking about not thinking, and not feeling. Here she was, sitting with a counsellor, neither of them saying anything. And yet, somehow, somehow it felt like what she had to do. Or was it need to do? She didn't know. Again, it felt too complicated to try and think about. Her thoughts drifted to her eating, how was she going to control it? How do you control an urge to do something that has been such a part of your life for so long, particularly when you know part of you really doesn't want to change? It suddenly all seemed too huge, too overwhelming to think about. And it felt threatening. She'd had quite positive days, but they were not in her mind now.

She wanted to say that she didn't want to change. And yet, just thinking of saying it, she felt she'd want to then say, "but I know that's not the answer". She just felt stuck, wanting to change, not wanting to change, wanting control, feeling she had to lose what was her control which meant gaining control felt like losing control . . . And her head began to spin trying to think about it, so she stopped. It was all too confusing. She had to keep it simple, somehow. Simple. What did that mean? She shook her head, still lost in her own thoughts, her own internal process.

Ginny noticed Carol shaking her head and responded, acknowledging what she was witnessing.

'Leaves you shaking your head.' She spoke softly, again not wanting to disturb Carol's process and yet seeking to communicate her empathy and her presence.

Silences can be profound experiences within counselling sessions. I have read chapter and workshop headings: 'working with silence'. No, it should be *'working with silences'*. The plural is important. There are many forms and qualities of silence. Each has its own meaning to the client and the counsellor needs to be sensitive to this. Sometimes it is appropriate and therapeutically helpful to say something to affirm the counsellor's presence, or that they have noted something of the client, and at other times what is needed is for the counsellor to respect the client's choice to communicate silence.

Carol continued shaking her head, but now it was in acknowledgement of what Ginny had said. She took a deep breath. Her head felt like it was full of gluey cotton wool. She closed her eyes. She could feel the discomfort in her throat. The medicine from the doctor had eased it, but it hadn't gone away, and eating, drinking, feeling tense, would all make it worse again. In a way she felt like she could just sit there forever, unable to get up. Unable to move. Just be stuck in the chair. And at the same time she knew that she couldn't stay like this. Yes, this was how she felt, her head felt heavy, her whole body felt heavy as she continued to sit in the chair. It felt like the slightest movement would take so much ..., too much, effort. She wanted to go to sleep. But what good would that do? She yawned again, and this time it left her feeling slightly less hazy. She blinked a couple of times and looked across at Ginny, who was sitting quietly, watching her, looking concerned. She saw Ginny acknowledge her look. Carol would normally smile but she simply didn't feel like smiling. In fact, she felt herself tighten her lips, and she noted that Ginny did the same, and nodded slightly. Yes, she can tell that I am in no place to smile.

What did Ginny know about her struggle? She seemed to be able to understand. But did she really understand? Did she? She certainly listened, certainly seemed to be able to hear what Carol was saying, and that felt important. But the thought that was with Carol was to do with whether Ginny really understood what it was like. Carol assumed that Ginny would have heard similar things from other people, so maybe that was how she knew. But that wasn't the same as knowing from your own experience. She wanted to know how much Ginny knew, really knew. It suddenly seemed very important.

'Have you had a problem like mine?' Carol looked steadily into Ginny's eyes. She didn't want some half-arsed response, some fobbing off. In fact, she didn't expect that of Ginny, and the moment she finished asking the question she felt her own unease.

Ginny listened to what Carol was asking of her, and she could see from the seriousness of the expression on Carol's face that right now, in this moment, this was an important question, and one that she wanted an answer to. It didn't feel like the kind of question to which you might empathise with the client's need to ask the question. The client *did* need to ask it, that was why she *was* asking it.

'No.' Ginny didn't elaborate. She saw no point in justifying herself. Her response was authentic and said without hesitation.

Sometimes a question is demanding an exploration of the meaning for asking it, but at other times it is direct and demands an honest response. The counsellor has to make a decision. What is the tone of the question? And yet they cannot dwell too long, to do so could imply hesitation and indicate that the counsellor is having to think how to respond rather than simply responding. Where a direct question is demanding of a direct answer it should be given, clearly and directly.

Carol nodded. 'But you seem to sort of understand.'

'I want to understand how it is for you.'

Carol nodded again, taking in Ginny's response, and processing it in her own way. She wants to understand how it is for me. OK, that sounds fair enough. But can she?

'It's shit, that's how it is for me. It's shit, I hate it, I want it to go away. I want to get on with my life and not have to think about ...', she was going to say "eating", but didn't, because actually that wasn't what had come to mind. Something else had come into her thoughts.

'Not have to think about?'

'Trying to feel comfortable with myself.'

'Trying to feel comfortable with ..., yourself?' Ginny could only reflect back what Carol had said, not fully understanding what she actually meant, what experiences were urging her to say what she had said.

'With *who* I am.'

'*Who* you are?' Ginny conveyed the same emphasis that Carol had placed on her use of the word "who".

'Who you are.' Carol shook her head. She felt herself playing with the words, turning them around. Who you are. Who are you? Are you who? Who am I? What am I? Where am I? Questions that felt like they could go on forever.

'Here I am, nearly 29 years old, spending my evenings trying not to eat. I mean, it's crap. Isn't it?' She took a deep breath and raised her hands to her face, rubbing her eyes. 'It's crap. And it's got to change, hasn't it?'

'You want the crap to change.'

Carol lowered her head and was taking a deep breath. She knew she had to find a way of getting herself out of what she was feeling. She looked up. 'I've got to get a life, for fuck's sake. I've got to forget about the past.' She lifted her right hand in front of her chest, palm outwards, and made a motion of pushing something away. 'Forget about it. What's happened has happened. I can't keep carrying it around with me. I learned to binge, I had reasons, I needed control, I needed to make decisions in my life, but they were then. And I made myself vomit it because I had reasons, I didn't want to put on weight. I know all this.' Her right hand continued to move, now pushing down in front of her. 'I've got to ...,' her left hand had joined in. 'I've got to push it all away, not bury it, I know that, but not keep living it out. That's who I was, and who I still am, but it's not who I want to be.'

'Mhmm, the person you were, you want to push that all away,' Ginny moved her hands in the same way as Carol had done, 'and become the person you want to be.'

Carol took a deep breath. 'And I'm not sure who that is.' Carol spoke softly and Ginny had to listen hard to hear what she said.

'Yeah, you're not sure who that person is that you want to be.'

'But I have to find out. I like my work, I do have a good social life, I do, but when I'm on my own ...'

'When you're on your own.'

'That's the me that I don't want to be.'

'Don't want to be on your own?'
Carol shook her head.

> The client has connected with a really important feeling, a sense of not
> wanting to be on her own. This part of herself now expresses itself; words
> and emotions emerge. It takes Carol into an area of herself that enables her
> to connect strongly with what she wants in her life. It is important that she
> makes this connection, voices what she feels and that all that is expressed is
> warmly accepted and valued. A yearning at the core of Carol's being is being
> voiced. It needs to feel heard, acknowledged, validated and reassured.

'I want to be a mum, I think I'd be a good mum, I know what it's like to not be
heard as a child, not to be able to do what you want to do. I wouldn't do to my
kids what happened to me.' Carol felt the tears in her eyes as she spoke, and her
throat felt constricted. 'But I don't want to be with someone like Tommy. And
I'm afraid that maybe I will be. It happened before. I don't want it to happen
again. They say you keep attracting the same kind of men, but I don't want
that, I-I really don't want that. How can I be sure? I mean, I have relationships – well, you know, a few weeks, if as long as that. But nothing too deep,
but that's what I want, but I don't trust myself, that bastard destroyed me.'
Ginny guessed Carol was talking about Tommy, 'desperate for a deep relationship, that will feel *good*.' Ginny knew that Carol hadn't said it quite like that
but this was what she was understanding and therefore she conveyed it back
to Carol.
'Yeah, yeah, something deep and good, someone I can feel at ease with, you
know, not some bastard that demands all kinds of crap from me. I don't want
that, I don't need that. I just want . . ., and I just want babies. And I know I
don't need a relationship for that. But I don't just want that, I want to have a
family, be part of a family.' Carol was aware of a heavy-hearted feeling. What
she was saying seemed so far away from her reality. So far away. And yet, her
feelings were so strong. Yet she knew she didn't trust herself and, if in doubt,
she knew she'd pull back, or pull out of a relationship. Well, she realised that
was important, part of her own self-protection. But it could be a problem too.
'You really want that, don't you, to be a part of a family?'
Carol nodded, and she could see in Ginny's eyes how much she was touched by
what had been said. Ginny's eyes were moist and Carol was aware that her own
eyes were watering again. She felt suddenly accepted, in a new, deeper, different kind of way. She swallowed and continued to speak. 'That's what I want.
I don't want the years to go by, Ginny, I really don't. I know people want to be
free and do their own thing, well, yeah, so do I, and I have been, but I want to
have children, have a family, I can't tell you how much. It's not something I
talk about, not something I try to dwell on, it makes me sad. I feel like it'll
never happen. I won't meet the right person. And, anyway, would someone

that I'd want to be with really want to be with me, some messed up bulimic woman? I wouldn't, why should they?'

'You're saying you wouldn't want to be with you, so you don't think anyone else would?'

Carol nodded.

Ginny thought of Lisa, whose presence albeit only as a friend – and Ginny was aware that that was an assumption on her part – sort of contradicted in some way what Carol was saying.

'I don't know, I don't know how to . . . , I was going to say that I don't know how to feel loved. I'm not sure if that's what I mean. But I feel mixed up, messed up. What is love? What is it, really? How do you know when it really is? I thought I loved Tommy, and in many ways I did, and parts of him I sort of still do I think, but other parts of him were a nightmare. I'm sure you can't love everything about someone, that's for fairy stories, I guess, maybe, but to love someone and not to feel that there are parts of them that will damage you, hurt you. I may not like everything, but someone who's caring, respectful, who's willing to share things, do things together, that's what I want.' Carol was looking at Ginny, the eye contact was strong and steady. 'That's what I want.' Carol shook her head as her thoughts and feeling slid back into her previous focus. 'And I have to stop thinking about food, and eating to feel good, and then throwing it up.' She shook her head. 'It gets me nowhere. I-I need to get a life, I mean that, people say it, and you think, "oh yeah", but I mean it, I need to get a life.' She thought of Lisa, she was such a good mate, and in a way she also felt that somehow maybe being in a relationship might threaten that. She didn't want to lose her friendship with Lisa, it was too precious, and maybe another reason not to get into something deeper with someone else.

'That's how it feels, it feels like you need to get a life.'

Carol felt stiff and stretched her back. 'I don't know how I do it though, other than, well, do different things, maybe meet different people. And I need to cope better with being on my own. I can't just eat. But I can't just go on feeling like I have recently. I know that as well.'

'Mhmm, coping with being on your own, that sounds like a big one?'

Carol thought for a moment as an idea suddenly came to her mind, something she hadn't really seen before, and yet it somehow made so much sense.

Ginny noticed the change of expression on Carol's face. She looked as though she had suddenly seen something, a kind of eureka moment, or "aha moment" as some refer to it.

'When you said that, I went back to childhood, and I was alone, I mean, as a teenager I was, I felt alone. I mean I wasn't alone, my parents and brothers were there, but I was alone because no one really was there for me, at least, it didn't feel like they were. They didn't feel like they wanted to hear me, so I was sort of alone. And my brothers I think got more attention, as well. They certainly had more freedom than I did. And I was sort of alone with Tommy. I mean, I was, having to cope with him, and the times waiting for him to come home – they were the worse. That was an awful aloneness.' She paused, as another idea came into her mind, 'do I eat to control feeling alone? I was OK when I left home, when I was in the flat with the girls. But then, I didn't feel alone the same then. I sort of don't feel so alone when I'm with Lisa although I can have my bad days. But maybe that will change. If I don't feel alone, with all the thoughts and feelings that come with that, then maybe I won't feel the need to binge? Does that make sense?'

Ginny nodded. 'What you are saying makes sense to me, that you feel that you eat on the feelings that are associated with being alone, feelings that were particularly awful when you were with Tommy, but which go back to childhood.'

What Carol has said is important to her, emerging spontaneously from within her. She needs to feel heard and understood. She needs the reassurance that what she is saying makes sense. It makes sense to her, but will it make sense to anyone else? Ginny is the "anyone else".

Carol nodded. Hearing it said again it somehow simply made sense. Yet she hadn't seen it like that before, at least not the way she was experiencing it now. Carol glanced at the clock and realised the session would soon have to end. 'OK, so this is helpful. It gives me a focus, something to work at. I have to either avoid being alone and/or make being alone feel OK. Yes?'

'That sounds like the two options, avoid being alone, and/or find ways to make being alone feel OK.' Ginny felt as though something had lifted. The heavier atmosphere that had been present for much of the session seemed to be dissolving. She felt lighter in herself as well. She smiled across at Ginny.

Carol smiled back. It felt good. She had something that helped her really make sense of things. Feeling alone, that was what she had to deal with. If that was driving her bingeing, then maybe the bingeing might settle down if she could feel more comfortable with herself? She hoped so. But she knew it was still a habit that she had to break. But it suddenly felt good sitting here, smiling, with Ginny smiling back.

Ginny had also noticed the time, and commented to the effect that the session was nearly over.

'It's been really helpful. Not easy, like struggling through a gluey fog. Thanks. This feels like the best session so far. I feel more positive, like I've found something out that gives me, I don't know, I feel sort of different.'

'Great, sounds wonderful.'

As they both stood up, Carol felt an urge to give Ginny a hug, but she also felt a resistance. She was older, she wasn't sure how she'd react. She didn't want to do something that might be wrong. She felt hesitant.

Ginny was still maintaining her attention on Carol, in her view sessions did not end as you stood up, the relationship remained, and she noticed the hesitant look on Carol's face, she looked troubled and given what she had just been experiencing she wanted to convey that she had noticed the change.

'You look hesitant, almost troubled, or maybe I'm misreading something?'

'No, no, I, er, well, I was feeling like I wanted to give you a hug and then I hesitated, wasn't sure if that was OK.'

'It's OK by me.' Ginny genuinely felt warmth for Carol, and a certain gladness that Carol had gained the insight that she had during that session. And for someone who struggles with being alone, who felt alone at home as a child, asking for a hug, and being given it, was probably enormously important. They hugged, and it was mutual, both women seeking to convey their appreciation for each other.

'Thanks. That felt good.' It was Carol who spoke first.

'OK?'

Carol nodded as she stepped back.

'Felt good to me too. So, see you next week.'

'I feel suddenly very different. I hope it lasts. It probably won't but it feels good. I've got to get myself coping with being alone, that's the first step. And I haven't forgotten the idea of a holiday I mentioned, was it last time?'

'I think so.' Ginny couldn't be sure, but she thought she remembered Carol saying something about it.

Points for discussion

- What stands out for you from this session?
- What role did the counsellor's unconditional positive regard play in the therapeutic process?
- Evaluate Ginny's practice as a person-centred therapist in this session.
- Discuss the development of Carol's experience of being alone and its psychological impact in terms of person-centred theory.
- If you were Ginny, what might you take to supervision from this session?
- Write notes for this session.

CHAPTER 5

Supervision session 2: the need to accept the whole client

'I need to talk about my work with Carol, she's having a tough time, finding aspects of her nature that are linked to her past coming back at her, so to speak. She's finding it hard not to slip back into the bulimic pattern, and has done on occasions. She's getting a lot of insight but the feelings that drive her need to binge and vomit are very present for her. It's distressing to listen to, she's fighting it, trying to overcome these patterns from the past, but they're hard to shift. So many mixed feelings around for her at the moment.'

William responded, noting his sense of Ginny's own experience of listening to her client. 'Carol's really caught between past and present, and that struggle must be having an impact on you, too.'

'It is. And I know that I have to keep offering her the therapeutic conditions, and that's not too difficult really. I mean, I am aware of what I feel for her, and I do feel warmth for her. And I know nothing is assured, but she's trying to make changes that she wants to make, and there is part of her that is fighting it.' Ginny shook her head. 'That's what's difficult, and I know that as a person-centred counsellor I need to hear all parts of Carol, that which wants change, and that which doesn't. They both need to feel heard and understood, and perhaps more so the part fighting against change, the thoughts, feelings, the beliefs linked to her sense of not having control in areas of her life, and of feeling alone. Both of these have emerged in the sessions, and quite powerfully so.'

'The part of her that doesn't want to change ...'

'... the part that is clinging to the bulimic behaviour, that part of her must be terrified of losing control. This is what is so challenging in this work, that we need to offer out empathy, warm acceptance to those parts or aspects of our clients that we can see are driving them to do damage to themselves. The human-being in me, the woman in me, wants to yell, "stop", but I know I can't, and that it wouldn't be the answer. Carol has to make her own choices, her own decisions, and I need to offer her – and particularly the part of her that does not want change – at least as much unconditional positive regard and empathic understanding as the rest of her.'

William nodded, 'and that is a challenge to us as person-centred counsellors, and you find it so as well.'

'I do. And yet I sense movement. I do see her making sense of herself, slowly recognising patterns, traits. I see her connecting with painful feelings and releasing them to some degree. I am optimistic and yet . . .'

'And yet . . . ?'

'Well that's it, isn't it? The unknown? What will happen? Carol has shown to herself that she can make herself not binge and vomit, but now it is about sustaining it, and she has identified how feeling alone is a major trigger for her to binge.'

'Mhmm, being alone leaves her with the urge to binge. How is that for you?'

Carol nodded and thought about her own reactions to what Carol was describing in the previous sessions. 'I can see it. It makes sense. It's deep-seated, back to teenage years, and then exacerbated by the violent and abusive relationship she had with Tommy. He really undermined her self-esteem, and she is struggling with that, but she is struggling, she's not giving up.'

William listened and noted that he had not heard Carol say much about her feelings and how it was for her listening to Carol and conveying the therapeutic conditions. 'So, Carol is battling with herself, her thoughts, feelings, behaviours, and I am wondering how this impacts on your congruence, your empathy, your unconditional positive regard towards her?'

'Like I say, I do feel for her. And as I say that I wonder to myself what I mean?'

William moved his head, conveying curiosity and inviting Ginny to say more.

'Well, it's like, I do feel for her, but I feel for the part of her that is struggling, and I guess what I am saying is that I find it harder to feel for the part of her that does not want to change.'

'The part that is afraid of being alone . . .'

'Terrified would probably be more accurate. And it's like I struggle to feel . . . ,' Ginny paused. 'No, I do feel that terror, I do have a sense of what that part is feeling, and I can feel unconditional positive regard for her within that experience, but it is then hard to feel the same when I know that part is driving the bulimic behaviour which in turn is doing her physical damage, and is in a way making the behaviour more firmly established. And that makes me then think that maybe I'm simply not accepting of her behaviour.'

'Not accepting of the fact that she does binge eat and vomit?'

'It's . . . , no, no, it's not that, not exactly.' Ginny paused. 'It's more that I can accept her need to do that, I can, I can see how it evolved, how it made sense. But, it's like I can accept the behaviour, and, yes, I think I can warmly accept it. I don't feel critical of her bulimia – that would be extremely unhelpful and I'm not there. But it's more the part of her that is driving or urging the behaviour, that's what I find it hard to warmly accept. I can understand it, it makes sense. She has done what she needed to do to have some psychological sense of control, to actually feel and experience control in a very tangible, and indeed physical, way. I know that. The terror she must have experienced waiting for Tommy to come home and start beating her, not knowing what she did that was wrong, beginning to believe that she could never get things right.' She shook her head. 'I don't think society has a full enough appreciation of the psychological and emotional damage that domestic violence has on people, not to mention the physical damage as well.'

'You sound passionate in what you say, Ginny.'

'I am. I am. I hate seeing any woman having to deal with this kind of nightmare experience. And I know men are victims as well.' She paused, her thoughts moving to earlier in Carol's life. 'I suppose, well, I mean, I can understand why Carol used food as a way to try and experience control and to sort of try and fill herself up, and then get rid of it to keep her weight under control. I can see it. And maybe, in a way, what I find harder to feel accepting of – no, that's not true. I don't accept Tommy's need to behave how he did towards her, and I don't want this to sound like a comparison, although it sort of is, but I find it hard to understand how Carol, as a teenager, and probably younger, could feel so alone. Seems like she was really controlled in that family. Her younger brothers seemed to fare differently, and particularly after Carol left home. Carol was a few years older than them, can't remember the age gap now, but it was significant.'

'You are saying that you find it harder to accept how Carol was treated as a child – maybe harder isn't the right word, but let's say you acknowledge that it is hard for you to accept that.'

Ginny nodded. 'I mean, OK, there are some bastards out there that treat their wives, partners atrociously. I know that.' She took a deep breath. 'And the trouble is, of course, there are parents who do the same, and maybe it doesn't always have to be so dramatic in order to have damaging effects. I suppose it's because children are more impressionable, are still developing, are learning about who they are, how they should be, all that kind of stuff. I can somehow just see how in a way Carol was set up for what happened with Tommy, I mean, not purposely, but as a victim of her upbringing. When the abuse started with Tommy then she reverted back to the only resource she knew, if you like the "configuration" within her self that was the bulimic behaviour – no, that's too simplistic, but something like that – that part reasserted itself. I was going to say bringing with it all its attendant thoughts, feelings and behaviours, but that feels back to front. Maybe it's more that she was put in a place of feeling very alone and out-of-control, and that triggered the behaviours that she associated with having those kinds of feelings.'

'It's not easy to be clear, but it's a matter of what triggers what.'

'And it has to be the feelings that were natural human responses to what she faced with Tommy, happened to be linked to, connected, I don't know what words to use, but in some sense brought with them a return to previous patterns of behaviour, and no doubt thoughts, linked to control – hence the bulimic behaviours coming to the fore once again, only this time they seem to have become more persistent, presumably because of the damaging effect Tommy had on her. The feelings are still present and alive and so the behaviour is hard to break.'

William nodded, 'yes, the feelings remain present, the need for control, the discomfort of being alone, yes?'

'She also talked about wreckage. The previous session to the last one had come to mind, 'feeling like she was picking her way through wreckage, but that she was, is, the wreckage. She talked of feeling "fucked up" as well. I think that she has been badly affected – I don't like the word damaged, but it does sum it up. And in a way, well, if you think about wreckage, and imagine you have to piece things back together, it's going to be hard sometimes to know what is what, what goes where, and maybe even whether what you find is something you want to remain a part of you.' Ginny was shaking her head and sitting tight-lipped as she thought about what she had just said. Yes, she thought, Carol is trying to make sense of who she is, trying to make sense of the parts of herself, the often conflicting parts, pulling her in different directions, feeling needs to satisfy, emotional, psychological, physical needs. The need to maintain a certain appearance; the need to feel in control; the need to try and avoid feeling alone. As she thought about these things Ginny could feel her own emotions becoming more present, and a certain softening of her feelings towards Carol. No, that wasn't the right word. It was more that perhaps she could feel more able to accept all the parts of Ginny, the different behaviours. They all had their place. They had all developed for reasons. They did all help her to maintain the presence of certain psychological experiences that she needed. And it had helped her survive, but there was damage, and now she was picking through that wreckage of herself, of her own life experiences, trying to in a way re-assemble herself, and to do so within a therapeutic climate of unconditional positive regard, empathic understanding and authentic being.

William had heard what Ginny was saying and now respected the silence that had developed. Clearly, Ginny seemed lost in her own thoughts and William chose not to disturb that process. Nothing was ever simple, or so it seemed. So much complexity. So much inter-connectedness within people's psychological landscape. Any significant change in one area and the whole system had to adjust. That was how it was. And this was major change. Dealing with what she had experienced went to the core of Carol's being, to her identity, who she was, at least, who she had become.

His own thoughts took him to the recognition of how the person-centred approach placed a certain primacy on the relational experience, of the counsellor working with the whole person of the client, or at least with as much as the client was prepared to bring into the therapeutic relationship. And it reminded him – although he did not need reminding – that eating disorders were so often an outer symptom of an inner something, a need, a hurt, a desperate attempt to satisfy a psychological imperative. And he knew that whilst changing the eating behaviour was one thing, as was how that eating was thought about, and what it meant, there was that need to go deeper – when the client felt ready for this – to re-engage with the underlying cause and, in the climate of the therapeutic relationship, discover perhaps a new perspective and an opportunity for the person to redefine themselves, but now in that crucial context of feeling unconditionally accepted and where authenticity was prized. He brought his thoughts back to Ginny, aware that he had drifted off. He maintained his silence, Ginny still looked very thoughtful.

'It feels like it's going to take some time, William, Carol has a lot to maybe face and, well, change if that is how it works out. I have to remember that my role is to offer the core conditions and to allow the actualising tendency to play its part. Well, that's a daft thing to say, it will play its part, regardless, but if I can help Carol to be more authentically herself, more truly aware of who she is and why, then maybe she will find herself making different choices naturally, spontaneously, to strengthen any fresh sense of self that may emerge.' She paused, and shook her head. 'So easy to say, so hard to accomplish.'

William nodded. 'So much is asked of our clients. They ask it of themselves, I suppose we do as well. Society has expectations that impact on what clients feel or think they should achieve, or how they should be like. So much pressure.'

'Pressure, yes. And I don't want to add to that pressure. The only pressure I want is to see that which comes from the actualising tendency as it seeks to – is it an "it"? – encourage a more fulfilling experience of life for the person.' Ginny paused again. 'It's not always easy to find the right words.'

'No, no, it isn't. I understand it as a kind of directional developmental process, not with a specific goal as such, but more as being the enhancing of the process of living.'

'I think Rogers wrote about "the good life" as "a process, not a state of being" (Rogers, 1967, p. 186) and that this experience of the good life was what was being sought. But that means being fully open to ourselves, our experiences, and feeling a genuine freedom to be. Carol is clearly not in that place. Her freedom to be is very much curtailed by her past experiences and the way that has left her seeing herself, experiencing herself, and the expectations that she now has of herself.'

Rogers wrote that "the direction which constitutes the good life is that which is selected by the total organism, when there is psychological freedom to move in *any* direction" (Rogers, 1967, pp. 186–7). It is the presence of incongruence within the person that curtails this freedom, leaving people to seek a satisfying life in ways that are driven by conditioned effects within the structure of self. As the person approaches a greater authenticity and fullness in their self-awareness and self-experience, then their capacity to achieve at any given moment an experience of the good life becomes more possible. But life is not static, it is process, and so such a state is not a final nirvana, but an on-going process of fluid responsiveness to events, circumstances and experiences.

Ginny continued for she was aware of how important she now felt about her own relationship with Carol. 'I feel somehow more aware of my need to be openly accepting to the whole of Carol, I can see that now out of what we have just been saying. I knew it, but I sort of know it a bit more clearly now. She needs to be as fully herself as she can be, and with less conditioning so that she can be authentically herself. But for her to be more complete and authentic, more openly a product of her own experiences, I have to warmly accept all of her. I am there to help her to become fully present, not so much to me as to herself. But I create – that's maybe not the right word – but I certainly seek to encourage a relational environment/experience in which the client, in this case Carol, may have the opportunity to more fully and authentically experience and be herself, and be supported in that ..., and accepted. So, what we've explored here I can feel has affected me. I think I had got tied up somewhere, caught in the complexity, seeing parts and not appreciating the whole, taking sides almost, which is counter-therapeutic from a person-centred perspective.'

William was listening and was nodding thoughtfully. What Ginny was saying rang true for him. 'Supervision can help us to entangle ourselves, even though we may not appreciate the actual process as it is happening.'

Ginny smiled. 'I'm not sure how I've got to feeling what I feel now, but I do feel that I can be more fully present for Carol, all of her. I suppose, in a small way, I am doing to myself what Carol has to do, untangling herself from everything that has impacted on her. And she has to pick her way slowly – back to the wreckage idea again – sorting herself, re-organising herself, her life. You can't rush it, can you?'

'No. And I think that's where a lot of people go wrong. We live in a quick-fix, solution-based world where people are expected to conform to treatment plans and fixed periods of work. Life is essentially not like that. All of that is human-made. Psychological processes flow at their own speed, and perhaps more freely when people are less pressured from outside – like if you try to push someone before they are ready then they are likely to resist, and then you have to take time resolving the resistance and its cause (the counsellor) before you can make progress on the real issue.'

The supervision drew to a close with Ginny feeling calmer in herself, but not complacent. She knew there was a lot of work to do and she felt more determined to ensure that she would be able to offer Carol a person-centred therapeutic relationship in which Carol, all of Carol, could feel welcomed and accepted, and hopefully, understood.

Points for discussion

- Evaluate William's responses and Ginny's use of the supervision session.
- Would you have raised other issues in supervision and, if so, for what reasons?
- What are your thoughts and feelings concerning the issues addressed in supervision?
- What are the unique features of person-centred practice as compared to other theoretical systems?
- If you were William, what might you take from this supervision session into supervision?
- Write supervision notes for this session.

CHAPTER 6

Four sessions of the client coming to terms with her life

Carol continued to attend the next four sessions, and continued to work at making sense of herself and her motivations to binge. She felt increasingly able to accept that her past experiences of relationship in her family and later with Tommy had made a significant impact upon her. Feelings were becoming clearer for her, and she could own them in a way that felt new to her. Her sense of being alone as a teenager, of not really being heard, of having to conform she could see had left her prepared to accept Tommy and his behaviour towards her for longer than she should have done. She had also begun to realise that the feelings she had still felt for him, even at the start of her therapy, were unreasonable and unrealistic, that they were simply the reactions of a person desperate for attention, for someone to be with her, who she could however fleetingly feel cared for by, however badly treated she had been for so much of the time.

Throughout the sessions Ginny had maintained her empathic sensitivity to Carol, and had continued to experience her own warmth and unconditional positive regard for her. It was an experience that she had which was quite natural and unforced. She felt very much as if she had been allowed into Carol's inner world of experience, gaining her own sense, from what Carol communicated to her, of how her life had been, and how it had left her thinking and feeling about herself and her experiences.

The image of sifting through wreckage had become something of a theme, in session five Carol had focused strongly on this.

'It feels so much as though I am having to work out what really is me. I mean, I know it is all me, but some of who I am causes me problems. And I know that my eating now, and then, is so much linked to how I viewed myself.'

At the time Ginny had felt a sense of appreciation of the insights that Carol was gaining for herself, and yet she was also aware of her own concern as to what changes Carol might be able to sustain to her eating pattern, and what resilience she would, or could, develop to avoid turning back to the bulimic pattern that had become such a feature in her life, and which had both psychological and behavioural meaning for her. But she set her concern aside. It was, after all, what she felt, and her role was to listen to and communicate her understanding of what Carol was experiencing, of what was more important to her.

Carol felt more fluid in herself at times, but not all of the time. As time passed she felt more able to think differently about herself and with that came an increasing openness to fresh insight and a readiness to question herself. At times this felt extremely risky, and at other times it felt much more natural. It led her to realise how much her sense of being alone left her struggling to feel more fluid. She could feel herself shutting down when she felt herself at risk of having to face something alone, or when she re-connected with feelings and memories from those periods in her life when she had felt it so acutely. At those times she became more fixed, stuck in those old familiar patterns. And, yes, at times she had binged again, but not as much. As she began to recognise more clearly the feelings, thoughts, the way of being that she felt emerge within herself in relation to the bingeing, she began to realise that they may be part of her but they weren't all of her, even if it felt like they took over. This became very important as she realised increasingly that she wanted to become more established in that aspect of herself that was not associated with her bulimic behaviour. She knew that, and had known that in her head before, but now the realisation had extended and was somehow more centred in her feelings, her desires, it felt as though it had shifted to a more central aspect of her nature.

She became increasingly angry – and not only towards Tommy. Anger also became more present towards her parents. She found herself wanting to have less to do with them, but that then also brought the threat of being alone back into the picture. She felt trapped. This became a theme in session six. 'I'm trapped, Ginny, I can feel it. I want my own space, and I had that, and I can still feel that I want that, in a way it has become more present again, but I don't want to lose my family either. But I don't want to, oh I don't know, it's hard to put into words.'

Ginny had nodded, unsure herself as to quite what Carol was trying to say, and had conveyed what she was experiencing and hearing from what Carol had said, hoping that perhaps it might help her to clarify her own thinking.

'You want you own space, a sort of freedom from your family, but you don't want to lose your family either.'

Carol had responded, underlining the comment that Ginny had missed. It felt important to her. It was the one feature that she could grasp. 'It's the feeling trapped. I don't know what to do. I need . . . ,' she had shaken her head, 'I need things to be different. I need to free myself from how I feel, how I felt, towards my parents. I feel freer in my attitude towards Tommy. Somehow it was clearer with him, at least it is now. But it's my parents, and there's something about that which still makes me feel that urge to binge.'

That sixth session had then moved on to a focus on the actual eating pattern that Carol had been maintaining. She described how she was aware that the feelings of wanting to binge seemed to emerge more strongly when she felt she did not have any control, and that the more she thought about her current situation, she could feel she had no control and that urge to binge became more present.

'I can feel that split within me really acutely sometimes. I can feel that feeling of, well, it starts with me feeling I have no control, but then it becomes a feeling of being trapped and it can then get out of control. I can feel it happening and I try to divert my focus – without eating, that is. A phone call, that's the best, someone to talk to, to get my focus off myself, or to get out. Lisa has been brilliant. But I know that deep down I wish I could talk to my mother about things. But I can't. I've just never felt close to her, and I wish I could change that, but I can't.' Carol had felt sadness as she had finished what she had been saying. Yes, she had all kinds of feelings towards her parents, but she felt unable to talk to them. She was sure they wouldn't understand, and maybe wouldn't really try. Neither of them seemed particularly warm, both were so logical, so much in their heads.

'You wish you could talk to your mother – you look sad.'

'I am.' Carol had felt the emotion rising within herself and it had led to a release of feelings that whilst it had left Carol feeling emotionally drained, had also felt both timely and necessary.

'I want her to understand. I don't want to blame her – well, I do, some of the time, I want to blame them both, I want them both to know how it was for me, and how it is. Maybe one day, I don't know. But not now. Now it all feels too much. Now I have too much to have to handle, without that as well.'

Ginny had expressed her empathic understanding and Carol had continued, feeling a sense of relief that her own sense of not wanting to say anything at that time was accepted by Ginny. Somehow that had felt important, more important than she had expected. She didn't want to feel pushed. She wanted to feel free to make her own choices, her own decisions.

During the seventh and eighth sessions Carol had continued to focus on her current eating pattern, what was making it easy, and what was making it difficult, going over the events of the week. She had resumed keeping a diary of her feelings and it was increasingly clear to her how particular feelings left her at risk of bingeing. She talked about them in the session and that seemed to help reduce their impact. She realised that she could feel them but could make other choices, that that was what she was having to do and yet somehow she felt more aware of it.

Ginny noticed that Carol's tone of voice had begun to change. She seemed at times more authoritative. It was as though her hesitancy and uncertainty would diminish and a new side of her character emerged. It felt good to Ginny to hear this aspect of Carol, yet she remained careful not to convey extra warm acceptance towards that part, clear that she didn't want Carol to feel that Ginny favoured particular aspects of her nature. Ginny wanted Carol to choose her way of being based on what she felt to be most satisfying and fulfilling.

It became more clear during session eight when Carol had been exploring her feelings towards her parents. She was due to visit them over a bank holiday weekend that was coming up. She'd wanted to talk it through. She had been angry before, but somehow that had felt different. She felt much more in control, this time, and it wasn't simply anger. It felt different, but she did not know what word to use to describe what she was feeling.

'So, a weekend with them both, and my brothers will be there, happy families.'
Carol had spoken with an air of resignation.

Ginny was aware of her strong sense of how much Carol did not want to go.
It was her tone of voice and her facial expression.

'Sounds to me like you really don't want to go.'

'I don't, and yet I do as well. I mean, no, I don't, I'd rather go off and do something
else. I know that. I can feel that. So, yes, I guess I don't want to go, but it's not so
much not wanting to go as wanting to do something else.'

'So wanting to do something else, that's the really important factor?'

'I want to get away, you know, that's what I want. I just feel like I want time on
my own.'

Ginny had noted what Carol had said, it wasn't something she felt she had heard
Carol say before. 'Time to be on your own.'

Carol nodded, not thinking about it in the same way that Ginny had. Somehow, it
felt simply what she wanted. Work had been busy, she'd put in extra hours.
She'd been out a couple of evenings during the week, the previous weekend
had been hectic, and she felt exhausted. 'I want to close the door . . ., no, no,
that's not what I want, I want to go somewhere, get away, somewhere open,
get some fresh air, just get away.'

'Just get away.'

'Yeah, that's what I'd like, that's what I feel I want,' she shook her head, 'but . . .'

'But?'

Carol had taken a deep breath, 'but I . . ., you know, I want to say that, well, to
question how it would be, you know? How would I handle it? But you know,
I'm not actually thinking that. I mean, I am now, but in a way because I'm
sort of amazed that I'm not thinking about that, I mean, not feeling anxious
about it.'

'You don't feel anxiety when you feel you want time to get away?'

'No. And that's different. And you know, I don't think I'd feel alone and I don't
think I'd want to binge because of it, and you know, even if I did, I mean, I
could come back, do something else, couldn't I?'

Ginny had nodded.

'So, you know, it's the thought of being back with my family for the weekend that
leaves me feeling like I'd want to . . .,' she smiled, 'that old bulimic me, I can feel
it, just waiting for an excuse.'

'Being with your parents feels like . . ., well, it leaves you aware of that "bulimic
you" waiting for an excuse to assert itself?'

'And that makes me feel so angry. I really feel that I have it more under control
now than I have for some time. I really feel as though I have achieved so much,
but the thought of being with them and, you know, it's there. And what's with
it is the thought that I won't be good enough. They didn't approve of Tommy
and had made that abundantly clear, and they blamed me for when it all ended
in disaster, I mean, not that I caused it but that I should have listened to them.
I hadn't done, of course, and wouldn't have done, on principle. But they were
right. And that's hard to say and to accept. I want to blame them. I do blame
them. But it was my choice, and it was a crap choice, and, yes, that was down to

me, but, well, if they disapproved then for me that was a reason to do it. That's how I became. It's still there. I don't want to conform and yet ...'

'You don't want to conform to your parents, and yet ...?'

'And yet ...' Carol let out a long breath, 'and yet they were right. But they weren't right about everything. And I've got to know the difference. I can't just react against them, that's what I did, and can feel myself still wanting to do. And that brings me back to the idea of wreckage, but in a different way.'

Ginny felt curious and it was reflected in her facial expression. 'In a different way?'

Carol nodded. 'Before it was like wreckage and I had to somehow piece it together, and decide what to keep and what not to keep. It's like some of the wreckage is right, things they said or did that were probably right. But other things weren't right. But I think I've still been seeing it as all being wrong because of my reaction against them. Something like that. I'm not sure I'm being very clear. It's been busy at work and I have had a hectic weekend. I'm feeling tired. And now I've got to visit my parents when actually I want time for me.'

Ginny had nodded and had sought to convey her understanding of what Carol had been saying. 'Your reaction to your parents makes it harder for you to choose what is right to keep because anything that is coming from your parents you don't want to accept? Is that what you mean?'

Carol had listened and it had sort of sounded right. She had felted frustrated, though. 'I wish I could just push it all away, gather it all up and set fire to it, make a huge bonfire and burn it all, get rid of it all and start again. That's what I feel like. It's like it's all too much of a headache to work out. Burn it all away and just be able to be me, a me that is comfortable with myself, that doesn't have to go on crazy eating binges, a me that can feel confident, that can do things because I want to do them, and that's because I really do, not as a reaction against anyone or anything. I just want to feel I can be me, freely me. And sometimes that's what I feel I'm working towards, and at other times it feels like such an effort. And at the moment I'm tired and it all feels like an effort.'

Ginny had responded, her response qualified by her feelings for Carol. Yes, she looked tired, she sounded tired. And yet she was gaining so much. Hearing her speak about wanting freedom to be herself, and what that meant. And the way she had spoken, it had felt so heartfelt. She smiled as she responded. 'That came from the heart. Wanting to be truly, freely, you. And at times you feel you're working towards it, but it's such an effort.'

Carol had nodded, 'yes, such an effort. But I don't have a choice. There is no way back, no path behind, not really. I know I have to keep moving forward.'

As that eighth session continued, Carol had become more and more aware that she didn't want to spend the whole of her Bank Holiday with her parents and brothers. She resented it, and she became increasingly aware of the force of that resentment.

'I'm not going to spend my whole weekend with them.' Carol had suddenly spoken and in a tone of voice that momentarily rocked Ginny. From amidst the struggle, the tiredness, the mixed feelings, the sentence had suddenly emerged with absolute crystal clarity.

'That sounds very, very clear. You are not going to spend your whole weekend with them.'

'No, no I'm not. I don't want to. I'm going to take some control here. I'm tired. I won't want to drive over Friday evening, I'll resent it, I won't enjoy being there. No, I have to do it differently, don't I?'

'You certainly sound very clear that you have to do it differently, and then I heard that hesitancy.'

'I'll feel guilty, I'll feel I should go, however I'm feeling, but it's madness. I'll be tired. I'm tired now, I'm bound to feel more tired by then. And to then drive nearly 150 miles, and the traffic will be crazy, bound to be. No, it's madness, utter madness. No, I have to tell my mother I'll come later in the weekend, after I've had some time for me. I know what she'll say, tell me how I can relax there, but I won't relax, I don't feel relaxed when I'm there.' She had shaken her head, clear that she had to make her own choices for the weekend ahead. 'I can see them, yes, and maybe stay over for one night, maybe two, but I want some time for me. I have things to catch up on in my flat, and I need to relax. I need it.'

'Mhmm, you need it.'

The session had drawn to an end with Carol clear that she was going to travel later in the weekend, she hadn't quite decided when, but she knew she had to do that. It wasn't just a wanting, it was a "had to". And she knew she had to be firm when she phoned.

Counselling session 9: the client experiences a revelation about herself

Ginny had been sitting before the session aware that she was wondering how Carol's weekend had turned out, and also aware that she knew that her curiosity was from within her own frame of reference, and it was for Carol to bring to the session whatever she wanted to talk about. Nevertheless, the strength of Carol's affirmation during that previous session had certainly made an impression, and so now she sat and wondered to herself whether Carol had asserted her needs, or not. She glanced up at the clock – it was nearly time for the session to begin. She closed her eyes and took a couple of deep breaths, bringing about a sense of stillness within herself, seeking to feel herself being clear and responsive.

Carol had arrived and was soon following Ginny back to the counselling room. 'So, how do you want to use our time today, Carol?'

'Lots to say. I'm feeling good.'

'Mhmm.' Ginny said nothing more, wishing to allow Carol the time and space to say what it was that she had "lots to say" about.

'I didn't go down to my parents until the Saturday evening, and I felt very positive about that. Yes, anxious as well. I mean, even though I explained that I was tired and needed some time, well, it didn't seem that it was what my parents wanted to hear. Told me, just as I anticipated, that it would be good for me to come down so I could relax. They just don't understand how tense I can feel when I'm there. Anyway, I ended up being pushed, I guess, into saying that I'd let them know how I was feeling on the Friday. They just didn't want to hear "no" about coming down that Friday evening. But I knew how I'd feel after work on Friday. And the thought of driving to them', Carol shook her head, 'no, there was no way I was going to do that. And I sort of decided that, well, I knew what I was going to do even if they weren't prepared to hear what I had to say.'

Ginny nodded. 'So, you knew in yourself what you had decided to do . . .'

'. . . yes, and I stuck to it. Well, I had to, I really was tired on Friday evening and I just knew all I wanted was to relax. Lisa and I met up for a pizza after work and then I went home, had a long, hot bath, and slept right through. And I needed it. I felt much more refreshed and did some stuff at home on the Saturday, time for me, and it felt OK. I knew I'd be heading off later and, well, I sort of put it off. I had thought of leaving early afternoon, but then it became mid-afternoon and actually it was about four-thirty when I headed off.'

Ginny was struck by the very relaxed manner in which Carol was talking. It wasn't that she hadn't seen her relaxed before, but somehow there was a difference. Hard to describe what it was, and she wasn't sure how much Carol was aware of it, but it was certainly something that was making an impression on Ginny.

'I'm really struck by how relaxed you are as you are telling me this. It sounds as though you took Saturday in your stride.'

'I did. Got done what I needed to do and headed off. I'd phoned them earlier in the afternoon, said I'd be there by seven-thirty. They were having a sort of buffet meal at home. I felt a little anxious in case I was going to be late, that was around. But, well, I know what they are like.'

'You know what they are like about people being late?'

Carol nodded, 'they like things to be how they have organised them. I mean, me not coming until the Saturday was a big thing, I really mean that. And I had to explain again why I'd come on the Saturday, and why I hadn't come first thing.' She shook her head and paused for a moment. 'Old feelings, they creep up on you, don't they?'

'You experienced old feelings creeping up on you?' Ginny sought to convey her understanding that Carol was talking about old feelings creeping up on *her*.

The client has made a specific connection that is important for her to communicate. It is very present for her. The counsellor acknowledges what has been said, offering an opportunity for further exploration should the client wish this. What was said previously has not been responded to. What the client said took her to the recognition that she then has. This is the place at which the client stops speaking, and it is in this place, or towards this place, that the counsellor then responds. The communication is therefore authentically alive to that which is present, and therefore therapeutically significant.

'Feeling controlled, having to comply with their demands. I felt that at home before I left. I could have done other things as well, but I stopped, knowing that I had to leave myself enough time so as not to be late. I could really feel myself getting anxious, and sort of rushing. I'd felt quite relaxed earlier in the day. But it sort of builds up, it did for me. And it's those sort of feelings that I know I could so easily binge on.' She shook her head again and looked down, 'So easily.'

'So easy to binge on those feelings.' Ginny spoke in a tone of voice that matched that of Carol's.

'It's like, I mean, I'm doing really well, I know I am. I know I'm feeling more in control now, I know that, and yet, I mean, when I experience those feelings again it makes me wonder, makes me realise just how much I'm still, well, at risk, I guess. I like to think that I'm sort of getting things together, but . . .' Carol was shaking her head again and could feel her heart thumping a little as she thought about those feelings. She could feel them now, as she thought about them. She wanted to be rid of them. She wanted to be rid of feeling that she hadn't got control. Control of what? The thought stayed with her. She took a deep breath. Control of her life. Control of what she did and when she did it. That was what she wanted, but she also didn't want to have to keep thinking about it like this. She had control now. She could do pretty much what she wanted. But it was like there was something inside her that still controlled her. A part of her but . . . , oh, she didn't know. It made her feel tired thinking about it.

Ginny had felt Carol lapse into silence. She didn't disturb it. She accepted it as a natural progression from what Carol had been saying and it somehow felt that for her to respond empathically to what Carol had just been saying would in a sense take her away, perhaps, from what had emerged for her within the silence. She sat, open to her own feelings of warmth for Carol who was saying she felt she was getting things together and yet there were these feelings, clearly linked to her parents' influence, that made her doubt or question this.

Carol's thoughts were back at her parents' home, and . . . It was the atmosphere, the tones of voice, the feeling of being humoured, yes, that's what it was, yes, being humoured. Carol needing to have her own space, even though it had upset her parent's plans. Humoured and . . . , what was the other word? She thought for a moment. Tolerated, yes, that was it, tolerated. She felt herself taking a deep breath. She was unaware that she had begun to shake her head again although Ginny noticed the head movement. It somehow seemed meaningful, there was a certain, well, it felt to Ginny like a certain resignation in the way Carol's head was slowly, and somewhat deliberately, moving from side to side.

'Makes you shake your head?' Ginny spoke softly, wanting to acknowledge the body movement but wishing to minimise the invasion of the silence.

'They just put up with me, I think. And yet some kind of criticism is never far away – what I wear, how my hair is, make-up, my work, it's like it's never good enough, never what they expected. And sometimes, sometimes I just want to tell them how it's been for me, I mean really tell them. But I really don't think they'd believe me.' Carol looked up, pain written across her face.

Ginny saw the expression and felt a wave of compassion 'Yeah, you'd really like to tell them, and it's so painful to feel they wouldn't believe you.'

'I can imagine . . . , I can hear my father, I know what he'd say. "That's a silly thing to do. We didn't bring you up to be like that." That's what he'd say. My mother, I don't know. She'd probably echo my father.' Carol was aware of the feelings she was now experiencing and she really didn't want to feel so heavy-hearted as she was. But it was there, and although she had asserted herself at the weekend, it had been at a cost. She knew that. But she hadn't binged or anything, well, she did when she got home – felt she needed to reward herself. She'd hit the chocolate on the Monday, given herself a boost, but she had contained it, and hadn't made herself sick. But she felt she might have done. She'd arranged to call Lisa when she had got back, but she did that after she'd got through a few bars of chocolate.

'That's what you can imagine, your father saying that it was a silly thing to do, your mother echoing what he had said.'

Carol sighed. 'Yeah, and I don't want to let it get to me. I suppose in their own way they mean well, but . . .'

'But . . . ?'

Carol shook her head and thought for a moment. It just didn't feel good being there with them, she felt always on her guard. 'It's like there's nothing that I can feel good about.'

For some reason it struck Ginny that this was a particularly important acknowledgement. She had no basis for this other than her sense that it was said with a lot of feeling. 'Nothing there that you can feel good about?'

Carol was looking down again, 'no'. She paused and looked up. 'And that's not how I want to be. And that's why I binged a bit when I got back. It did make me feel good. I didn't think badly about it. It was simply a case of knowing I needed something, something for me, something sweet, something that felt . . . , just felt good.'

'Something that just felt good, that was so important.'

'It was, it really was. It was like, "oh, now I can relax, now I can be me". I suppose, I mean, well, I'm trying not to binge but, well, it's what I did, and it wasn't that much and I didn't make myself sick. Thought about it but didn't. Funny that. Somehow I just didn't want to.'

'Thought about making yourself sick but didn't really want to.'

Carol nodded, listening to what Ginny said had given her time to stay focused on what she had said and how she had felt about it. 'Yeah. But I did control it, and that was good. But I sort of knew I was going to do it and I guess I sort of gave myself permission.'

'Permission to eat the chocolate?'

'And that seemed to make it OK. I mean, I didn't sort of battle with myself, and I didn't sort of feel out of control either.'

'Mhmm, so a sense that it was a controlled decision, a controlled act, is that what you mean?' Ginny thought she had grasped what Carol was conveying but felt she needed to check out her understanding.

'It was. It wasn't that I sort of blindly took off. It was like I sort of, I don't know, it's really hard to explain.'

'Hard to explain in words but within yourself you can experience a difference.'

Carol nodded. 'It really was different. And maybe that feeling in control, I mean, that's the weird thing, isn't it? I'd eat to feel in control, and then make myself sick, also feeling in control, but actually I was out of control. But I didn't experience it like that.' Carol paused as she reflected on what she had just said.

'You didn't experience it as being out of control, for you it had felt as though you were being in control.'

'Doing something that broke me free from their control over me.'

'Mhmm.'

'But I . . . , but it was different when I came back this time. I did feel in control. There was a time when I would have binged, well, I did, I know I did, and made myself sick, and it would have given me something, but this time, I mean, I sort of knew that it wouldn't and I sort of didn't need to. It was strange.'

'Strange to have those feelings of knowing you didn't need to?'

'I had control. OK, I binged on chocolate, but it wasn't uncontrolled. And because I knew I had control, that it was my choice . . . .', she paused again, 'yes, my choice, it really felt like it was "my choice", somehow different.' She shook her head again and frowned.

'There was somehow something different about your sense of it being "my choice"?'

Carol was in her own thoughts, "my choice", the two words seemed to strike a chord inside her. She knew how she so often had never felt that she'd been able to make her own choice as a child. Her thoughts then went to Tommy, her choice, crap choice. She wanted to make her own choice, but could she trust herself to make the right choice? That was the question that now bothered her. She wanted to make her own choice, and the chocolate was her choice, and, well, it seemed an OK choice. Hmm, control, the thought was back with her again. Control. I need to have control, OK, I need to make my own choices, OK, I need to feel that I can make . . . , yes, yes that was it. She spoke, 'I need to feel I have control in making my choices, and that I can trust that it is a good choice. I guess bingeing and being sick wasn't a good choice, and neither was Tommy, and yet they seemed to be at the time.' She stopped speaking and looked down.

Ginny didn't say anything, it seemed to her that Carol was still in her own process and did not want an empathic response distracting or disturbing that process.

'It's hard to trust yourself to make good choices when you know you've made crap ones, and you've had years of people – my parents – that you should do this, be like that, making you feel that their way is the only way. And then doing things simply because they were not their way. That's not the answer either, is it? And that's what I've been doing, and I have to make my choices, but I mean really my choices.'

Ginny was very much aware of the way Carol was speaking. There was a sense that she was processing her words as she spoke, or her words were expressing her process of making sense in her own mind what was happening. It felt very alive, very real, and had a sort of "tentative newness" about it, strange words to combine but they were what had come into her mind.

'Been making choices that you thought were yours, but were a reaction against your parents?'

'But when I make my choice, really my choice . . . , how can I be sure that it really is my choice?' Carol looked at Ginny, frowning, suddenly aware of a profound sense of not knowing within herself.

'When you make a choice, how can you be sure it really is yours, really is your choice.' Ginny spoke slowly.

'Freely mine, being free, that's an important part of this, being free.' She shook her head, 'I left home to be free, and, well, I was, sort of, but I was still being affected, wasn't I? I wasn't really free, was I? I was just reacting against and thinking that what I was doing was me being me, but it was me just not being them.' The sentence had flowed so easily from her lips, and yet it had so much meaning for her, so much relevance. It captured it, exactly, that was how it was, how it had been, and it had to stop, *had* to stop.

The client is indicating that she rebelled against the values of her parents by seeking a life that was in marked contrast. Within this was her bulimic behaviour. She has, one might say, introjected the value of control expressed through the control she manifests in her eating, however, she now recognises that in order to free herself from the values she internalised from them, she has simply reacted against and sought behaviours and experiences opposing those that her parents sought to impress upon her.

Either way, the values of her parents remain a significant influence, and now she is recognising this as she realises that true freedom for her would be to neither live out her parents' values, or live out their opposites, but to be able to freely choose what she wants for herself, free of these influences. This realisation can be quite shattering to the individual in the sense that they might only now be realising that who they are is still bound up with their parent's influence, and in some cases may leave the person with real uncertainty as to who they are, what values are truly their own. This is now a very significant phase in the therapeutic process.

Ginny nodded, maintaining eye contact with Carol. She noted the look on Carol's face, there was a sort of surprise etched into her face and yet there was also something of a look of horror as well. She looked stunned by what she had said. Ginny wondered whether to convey her empathic understanding of what Carol had said, or what was being communicated through her facial expression, or at least what she was reading into that facial expression. But she didn't want to sit thinking about it, but respond with the spontaneous warmth that she could feel within herself.

'You not being them, you look shocked.'

'I am. I mean, I sort of knew it but, well, I didn't as well. I mean, I . . .' She lapsed back into silence. ''Have I just been a me that was trying to not be them?'' The question was very present for her. She felt strangely numb, her arms were sort of heavy, she felt weighted in the chair. She could feel the frown on her face. 'Who am I?' The words came out quite quietly. Her facial expression had assumed a certain intensity, a kind of searching, and yet within that expression was now a kind of, well, a kind of shrinking back. That was exactly what Carol was feeling. It was as though she was pulling back, retreating away from what she had said. She'd heard herself say the words but she didn't want to know them, not really. She wanted to be herself, but who was she? Who was Carol? What did Carol really want? She had begun to shake her head slightly.

'Who is Carol?' Ginny waited, aware of her own feelings of sensitivity as she had spoken. There was something so poignant in the atmosphere, a stillness.

The words seemed to go right inside her, gently, not like a knife, they sort of just permeated her being . . . Her being. Well, yes, it was her, but still that who was she, who is this person wondering who Carol is? Had to be different, had to be. But had to have control, had to. And now . . . ? What now . . . ? She felt still inside herself. A quietness. Who was Carol? The person who behaved in all the ways with which she was so familiar? The person who had so much tried to be free, but who had really only taken her cue from her past, breaking free only to become shackled to a need to be different, to rebel, to be herself . . . , except that she hadn't been herself at all, not really. She didn't know who ''herself'' was.

Carol looked at Ginny. 'I don't know.' She frowned. 'I don't know . . . , I really don't think I know. The Carol who binged, who tried to break free of all the control, who made herself sick to control her weight . . . , who was that person . . . is that person?' She shook her head. 'Me, but not me. Yes, me, but . . .' She lapsed into silence, taking a deep breath as she did so. 'What's happening?'

'What's happening?' Ginny responded with a questioning tone, wanting to understand more fully what Carol was experiencing.

'It's like I feel I'm waking up, and it feels very new and strange. It's like something's, no, everything has changed. What happened?'

'You've awakened in some way, and it feels as though everything has changed?'

'I don't need to be how I have been, do I? I mean, I really don't.' Carol paused for a moment. 'I really don't. It's strange. It's so sudden. I couldn't see it, but now I can. I haven't been me, not really me, just trying not to be what they wanted me to be. I took control, but I got out of control. Eating, bingeing, living my own life, what I thought was my own life . . . How far does it go? There must be things I have done for me, really for me.' She looked down and shook her head. She felt quite disorientated, and yet it felt OK, it felt strangely OK. 'Something's shifted, something big. I don't really know what it means, but something has happened. Listening to you, when you said about how could I be sure it was my choice, it was like I heard you, me, in a different way. The words went through me. I knew that I couldn't be sure, I didn't know. I thought I did, I knew I did, and then I didn't.' She shook her head again, 'and now it seems as though I've got a lot to make sense of.' She smiled weakly as she looked up.

Ginny nodded, 'a lot', and smiled back.

Carol was taking a very deep breath. She closed her eyes for a moment, opening them as she realised she felt a little dizzy. 'I need some water.' She reached over to the glass. 'I don't need to eat, or not eat. I don't need to make myself sick. I don't need to feel in control . . . , well, maybe that's going too far, but it feels like I'm just in a different place.' She felt puzzled, and it was expressed on her face.

'In a very strange and different place.' Ginny was reading Carol's facial expression, but used the word "strange" because it was in her mind because Carol had used it herself previously.

'It is strange, and I can't make sense of it, but it feels like there is a lot to make sense of. And even as I say that, it somehow also suddenly seems so simple. It's been so complicated, my life, me, who I've been, how I've been. I don't need that, I really don't. It's like although it's strange it somehow feels sort of easier, in some way.' She nodded to herself, allowing her thoughts to flow on. Easier. At ease, maybe at ease with herself? She did not know, but she was so very aware of the shift that had suddenly occurred and so unexpectedly. She felt she needed some quiet time to just be with herself – be with herself. She felt herself want to smile. Almost like needing to get to know herself, which in a way seemed silly, and yet . . . She felt herself taking another deep breath, she didn't know what else to say. It felt as though, for the moment at least, there was nothing to say. She needed to just stay with what she was experiencing. 'I need to just sit with this for a while, is that OK?'

Ginny nodded, widening her eyes slightly as she did so, and smiled. 'Sure, just be with what is happening.'

Carol sat, the stillness remained, and the quietness. She really didn't need to be the way she had been – not that she wanted to completely stop being the person she had been. But she just knew, inside herself, that there wasn't such an urgency. She hadn't really thought about it like that before, but now the thought was with her. She felt relaxed, under no pressure. Pressure. That was something she was used to feeling. Being busy, filling her life up, trying to avoid too much time on her own . . . Filling herself. Yes, she'd done a lot of that. How was she feeling now? Empty? No. But not full, just . . . , she wasn't sure how to describe how it felt. She felt sort of, well, just OK. Just OK? No, not "just" OK. She felt good. She felt OK. She shook her head slightly and felt herself frown. The stillness seemed to fade a little. She didn't want to lose it. She was thinking too much and it was unsettling the stillness. She didn't want it to go. Mustn't think too much, she thought to herself. Another deep breath. It felt good, she felt good, but she didn't want to have to think about it.

Ginny sat and maintained her focus, and her attention on Carol, not wishing to intrude. She could hear the silence, it felt alive in her ears. She felt herself in total concentration, a sense of feeling quite absorbed into her experience of what was happening, into the silence, into the stillness. She didn't move, she didn't dare move. It somehow wouldn't have been right, wouldn't have felt right. It felt as though the slightest movement would somehow disturb what was present, would be like throwing a rock in a clear, still pool.

Carol looked up, took another deep breath, closed her eyes and looked down again. She nodded to herself, slowly. 'I think that maybe I have begun to find myself. Quite what that means, I don't know. But thank you. I don't really understand what has just happened, Ginny, and maybe will eventually. Now I feel like I just need to go and be quiet for a bit longer, maybe for as long as I can.'

'Mhmm, preserve that quietness.'

Carol was nodding to herself again. The session drew to a close and Carol headed home. Ginny sat back and pondered on how the session had left her feeling.

Points for discussion

- How has the session left you feeling? What has happened? Discuss in terms of person-centred theory.
- What enabled Carol to enter into a different 'place' in herself?
- What part might her experience in relation to the weekend with her family have played in this?
- Evaluate the counsellor's therapeutic responses and way of being as a person-centred counsellor.
- What would you take to supervision from this session?
- Write notes for this session.

Reflections

A couple of weeks have passed and Carol is sitting at home pondering on what has happened over the weeks she has been in counselling. She talks about her experience.

'It's not what I expected, none of it was. I really expected that I'd have to talk about my eating all the time, but it just wasn't like that. Yes, we did, of course we did, but somehow . . . , no, I was going to say that it wasn't important, but of course it was. And yet, well, it wasn't the real problem, and it still isn't, although it is.

'That stillness faded, but it has come back as well. But I can get so caught up in my life, in my work, I sort of lose it and have to remind myself. That session where it happened, it just left me thinking about so many things, and not wanting to think about anything – at the same time. It was strange. But I can feel, now, that I am different. Not all of the time, and I feel old anxieties arising as well, but I seem to be sort of able to feel different about myself. I'm still getting used to it.

'That urge to be in control isn't there like it was. I still eat chocolate, but it's a different experience, somehow. There's not that *need*, somehow. I feel sort of lighter – I don't mean weight-wise, but somehow a deeper lightness, it's hard to describe. I guess it's something you have to experience to sort of know.

'Ginny sits and listens, and keeps listening. It feels like that's all she does, and yet I know she doesn't. She's there, somehow . . . , and it makes me frown thinking about it because I don't understand what it is that she does, but it sort of makes me feel different. At times I wonder how I might have been if my mother had been like her. But I know that she isn't, but I do wonder. Maybe I'll mention that sometime, I don't know.

'I feel different about my parents. Not all of the time, but there's something new in me now. That urgent need to be a particular way, it was though I wasn't aware that that was how I was. I'd just drifted into being how I was. Quite oblivious to it, wrapped up in it. I guess that's what happens. So intense. Never really thought of myself quite like that, but I was, and I guess I can still be – well, I know I can, but it's like I'm learning another way as well now. It makes me smile. I'm sure I should be concerned, something happening to me that I have no control over. But I don't, not really. Yes, I wonder what's going on. And maybe I won't always feel like this, but I do at the moment and I want to explore this some more.

'Funny how counselling sort of grows on you. I'm becoming more curious about myself. I want to understand myself more. Whether I'm free of the bingeing and making myself sick, well, I hope so, but, well, I feel I have to watch myself. But be gentle on myself as well. Maybe it's OK to give myself permission to have the chocolate. It's not the chocolate, or anything else that's the problem. It's how I feel, and how I feel about myself. If I feel crap then, well, I'm more likely to over-eat and, well, then I'd make myself sick. Haven't done that for a while now. I sort of miss it, though, in a strange sort of way. Haven't made sense of that. It's like part of me, it's sort of, I don't know, I guess when you do something for a long while it sort of becomes part of you. And yet I also feel a certain revulsion at the idea of making myself sick now as well. But there's that sort of sense that I could still do it, if I really felt like it. I could. And maybe that's because I know that I have. It wouldn't be new. But, well, I don't really want to think about that too much. I'd rather focus on getting my life together and having a good time, you know?'

It was around the same time that Ginny was also reflecting on the counselling process and her experience of being with, and working with, Carol. 'She's changed so much. She seemed to take a while to settle, but then, well, I think she was ready for change. People come along at different stages, and things can happen that move them along, sometimes within the therapy, but often in life. Sometimes it feels as though being in therapy almost acts as a kind of catalyst, forcing the process in some way. Maybe that's what it is, the actualising tendency finds maybe a new direction, for some people, maybe not for everyone, but somehow as a person works towards a fuller congruent experience of themselves, well, maybe they do in some way sort of attract experiences in life that sort of have meaning for that process. Maybe. I don't know.'

'It's just that the weekend Carol had with her family, somehow that seemed to loosen something up inside herself. She'd already taken her own steps by travelling when she wanted, so something was already moving, changing, shifting. She seems more fluid now, more open and accepting, and yet it has been a relatively short space of time. Whether what has happened is sustainable, I don't know. I really don't know, but it sort of feels like it may be. But, well, who knows what will happen next in a person's life? We never know what is around the corner.

'I feel good being with Carol. She has a sort of energy about her. Yes, she's had some difficult experiences in her life, a lot of conditioning in childhood, and a physically and psychologically abusive relationship. I sort of expect that maybe there will more to emerge, perhaps. It feels a bit like the stillness that sometimes follows a storm at the moment, but is the stillness permanent? Probably not. It rarely seems to be. I am sure thoughts and feelings will emerge for Carol if she continues with the therapy. She certainly seems keen to do so.

'It has been quite interesting working with a client who is quite emotionally literate. Not everyone is. Many clients can be more silent, or be more limited in their use of language, particularly when it comes to expressing feelings. When that's the case, I have to work with what is being communicated to me. At the end of the day, it doesn't really matter how emotionally literate a person is – that's my belief, anyway – what matters is the relationship, and the way the client perceives that relationship and hears, feels, experiences the empathic understanding I am seeking to communicate, feels the unconditional positive regard I am experiencing towards them. And, of course, my being congruent, well, as fully as I can be at any given moment. Being open to being me, that's how I like to think about it. And my horizon continues to expand as well.

'I haven't said much about eating disorders, have I? Would I describe Carol as a client with an eating disorder, or who had an eating disorder? I don't feel comfortable with the language. And yet we have to use words to convey our understanding of a person's behaviour. And yet behaviour is so often the tip of a psychological iceberg. When we give someone a diagnosis it can so often sound like an illness. Yes, the eating behaviour may become problematic, as with Carol, but in a sense they are secondary problems to those that fuelled the need to develop that eating behaviour in the first place. Of course, in extreme cases, such "disordered" eating may be causing such chronic physiological problems that these become the primary problem and need dealing with, simply to preserve the person's life to give them a chance to then deal with the underlying difficulties. In other cases, the reverse is true. And as a person-centred counsellor I definitely want to trust my client to know what they need, and I also know that that trust is itself an expression, no, wrong word, has validity because it is present within a relationship, a therapeutic relationship, in which the attitudes and values of the person-centred approach are present.

'I enjoy the sessions, I hope they continue, and I feel sure that Carol will know when she needs to stop. I am not trying to cure her, make her better, "fix" her. I offer a relational experience based on certain principles, with the recognition of my client's capacity to seek a more full and congruent experience of themselves. Yes, for me the presence of the actualising tendency lies at the core of my practice. The discipline of person-centred working allows it to encourage, within the client, greater congruent experiencing. This has certainly been, and continues to be, the experience for Carol.'

PART 2

Mandy accepts that she is severely underweight

CHAPTER 7

Counselling session 4: client reacts to the counsellor's honesty, wants to leave and nearly passes out

Mandy sat in the chair in the counselling room feeling very quiet and withdrawn. She looked down and counted the patterns in the carpet. She didn't want to be there, and she didn't feel there was anything wrong to make her have to be there. She hated talking about herself – she hated herself, well, not all of herself, just her shape. She didn't understand the people around her who told her she was too thin, that she should put on a bit of weight, fill-out a little. That wasn't how she experienced herself. As far as she was concerned she just felt . . . , the words that always came to mind were, "like a lump".

It was her fourth session of counselling. The first she had found difficult, hadn't had much to say. She'd been referred to this place by her doctor. The man opposite seemed nice enough, seemed relaxed, not "suited up". She felt herself taking a deep breath. She wanted to be left alone, to be on her own, be how she wanted – needed – to be. That was how it had always been at home. She just wanted to be left alone.

Her doctor had talked a lot about how much she was damaging herself, how she needed to eat, make herself strong, put on some weight, that it would be good for her. Good for her! What did he know? Last thing she wanted. Why couldn't people see it how it was? Why couldn't they understand? She was *fat*, she could see it, feel it, why did everyone else ignore it? Why? She shook her head, momentarily lost in her own thoughts and frustrations.

The second session she had said a little more, though still hadn't wanted to say much. Again, there had been a lot of silences. Why did everyone think she had to change? Why did they think she was unwell? Strange, though, her counsellor didn't seem to be saying that. He seemed to accept her, well, he wasn't saying what everyone else said. Not yet . . . He seemed to let her have time to just sit, everyone else seemed to have so much to say, but he seemed to let her be. It was certainly different. She couldn't really make sense of it.

Ian sat and felt himself wondering how he would make a connection with his new client. In the first session he had explained about confidentiality and what counselling could offer. It had seemed to him that Mandy had taken it in. But she clearly didn't want to be there, didn't want to talk, at least, that was how she seemed to be. He recognised, of course, that he needed to take care with such assumptions. People were silent for many reasons and just because he interpreted it one way, however strong the feeling might be, did not mean that he was right or that he should voice his thoughts.

The third session had been a bit like the first – Mandy not saying very much, a lot of silences, which he had stayed sensitive to and had not interrupted. He had maintained his attention and focus, and felt sure that the warmth he felt for Mandy was an important factor in the process of establishing a therapeutic relationship. He knew that what he was offering couldn't be rushed. He had responded to her when she had spoken, and he had been attentive but he hoped not invasive, during the lengthy silences that had arisen. He imagined – again, he noted it as being his own internal process – that Mandy may have a lot to think about within herself, perhaps keying into particular thoughts or fears. Still, he had known it wasn't for him to speculate. He felt for her, though, she did look thin and quite pale, drained was the word that had come into his mind the moment he had seen her, drained, and yet there was also something strong about her as well, something quite intense. It was an impression that he had, but he knew he might be misreading his perceptions.

It would not be unusual for there to be silences in the first sessions of therapy, and different therapists will respond to this in their own way. Perhaps the client feels they have nothing to say, or don't want to acknowledge why they are attending. There may be a wish to deny to experience any awareness of the notion that they have an eating disorder. Or they may recognise it but it is too difficult to think or feel about. What does the counsellor do? It may depend on the context in which the counselling is taking place. In this case, the counsellor stays with the client's choice to be silent, and remains attentive to their frame of reference. Others may well more actively voice the fact of the problem area, particularly when referred specifically for this purpose. Marchant (2005) has pointed out how, in her own work with clients with anorexia, she has found it helpful in those silences 'to address the client's eating pattern quite openly and without shame'. She adds, 'for me it is something along the lines of if I can speak freely and openly of their anorexia, in the silence perhaps, and without judgement of my client, in this instance it is through this that I believe I can convey my acceptance of her entirely and hopefully she can begin to trust in a relationship with me'.

In neither of the first three sessions had Mandy said much about her eating, other than she was tired of being told what was good for her, and of how frustrating that was. She'd said a little bit about her parents, her brother and sister, both older than her and both having left home. She had begun to speak more as the sessions had proceeded and whilst to begin with she had looked very withdrawn, with very little eye contact, that had changed, or at least it had begun to change. But today she seemed to be somewhat withdrawn again, looking down. Ian just had this sense of distance. Not that there had been a sense of closeness. Now it was the fourth session and he was pleased that she had arrived. She'd said in the second session that she wasn't sure whether she wanted to bother coming, wasn't sure what good it would do, but she felt she had to. She had said in the third session, though, that actually it was OK being there.

For Ian, his intention had been to listen and understand what Mandy was experiencing. As a person-centred counsellor he was not there to tell her what to do. She was receiving medical care and monitoring of her physical condition. He knew others were encouraging her to acknowledge that her lack of eating was causing a health risk. At times he could feel that urge to say something himself, and he recognised it as coming from his own heart, his own sense of humanity, his own wish to help another person not cause themselves more physical distress when it could be avoided. And yet ... He also knew that his role was to offer that relational space, that opportunity for Mandy to be able to be herself, to feel heard and hopefully understood, to maybe risk revealing to others some of her innermost fears and motivations between her choice not to eat and to view her body in whatever way that she did. He sought to be attentive to her, and he felt he had been achieving this. Yes, there had been lots of silences, and he had acknowledged them and he had indicated that he was quite accepting of them if they were what Mandy felt she needed. He wanted her to feel accepted and acceptable for who she was and what she thought and felt. He knew that without that, there would be no therapy, not as he understood it. He knew that the relationship was key and that it took time and self-discipline to allow it to develop.

He looked across at Mandy, wondering how she might want to use the counselling session. 'So, how do you want to use the time today, Mandy?'

Mandy sat, still looking down. She'd heard Ian speak. His voice had sounded quite soft and she tightened her lips, not knowing quite what to say. She wasn't sure about counselling, and found herself taking a deep breath. She sort of felt good about coming in a way. She was a little surprised as she realised that was what she was feeling. It sort of felt like time to get away – get away from people telling her what to do and how she should be. What did they know? What did anyone know? Why didn't they understand? Why couldn't they see that she had to be really careful about what she ate?

The silence continued and Ian waited. He was OK with silence and, well, it was very much a feature of the relationship. He felt it was a relationship. He knew that contact and perception did not have to be extensive, that it could be quite minimal and yet there could still be therapeutic effect.

As he looked over to Mandy he did feel for her. It was a kind of sadness, but that wasn't quite the right word to describe it. It certainly wasn't pity, maybe more of a feeling for Mandy as a young person, a young girl, with a life to be lived ... He pulled his thoughts back. She was living her life, now, as she felt she needed to and it was for him to accept that. And yet he couldn't help experiencing a sense of wanting her to ... He couldn't quite grasp what it was that he wanted. It was sometimes difficult in silence to hold his focus. He was affected by his clients, they moved him and he was glad that they did. He wanted to experience this. He believed it was an important aspect of the therapeutic process. He needed to be affected by his clients, touched by their stories, their lives, yet more than that, be touched by them as persons, as fellow human-beings often trying to make sense of themselves, their lives, their choices. And sometimes not knowing what they wanted, who they really were, just wanting someone to try and understand them, maybe help them believe they could be understood.

These were not the thoughts in Mandy's mind. She didn't want people to understand her . . . , well, in a way she did, but she also had a strong feeling of "fuck them, what do they know?". That was how she felt a lot of the time, but beneath that there was a yearning to be understood, to be loved, cared for, accepted. No, for Mandy her main focus was control, feeling in control, being in control. She didn't want to lose that.

She still said nothing. What would she say? Her dad had been on at her again about eating. Her mum, well, she'd tried . . . Oh, what was the point. She was more interested in her friends, in going shopping, chilling out around town.

It had been the doctor's idea that she see a counsellor, someone at the surgery. Well, here she was. She continued to say nothing.

Ian felt OK with waiting, and he also wanted to be empathic to Mandy's clear decision not to say anything. Whilst he respected her right to silence, he also recognised that sometimes – and in his experience this was often true with some young people – there was a need to be a little more proactive and reach out. He didn't apply this to everyone, but sometimes he did experience a stronger pull to say something to establish connection. Was it for him to feel connected, though? Was it his need, or the client's? What did Mandy want? Maybe she did want to just come and sit and spend time in silence. She certainly had control of the session.

'You don't say a lot?' Mandy had looked up as she spoke.

'No, I suppose I don't.'

'You're the only one.'

'Only one, who . . . , who doesn't say very much?'

'Everyone else goes on at me. Like I've said before, they don't understand. I don't think they want to understand.'

'You don't think any of these people that go on at you want to understand you?'

'They all think I've got a problem, but I haven't.' She thought about saying more but realised she didn't want to.

'Mhmm, everyone else thinks you have a problem, but you don't.'

'What's wrong with them?'

'It feels like there is something wrong with them, they just don't see it the way you do, and you can't understand why.'

Mandy shook her head. 'Pisses me off.'

'Mhmm, you feel pissed off by the way they don't seem to understand, must be a real pain.' Ian added the last comment in. It wasn't exactly empathic in terms of what Mandy had said, but it was emerging from a wish to communicate his appreciation of how it must feel to be someone surrounded by people who don't seem to want to understand you.

'Yeah. They tell me I'm the pain, my mum, dad, my brother, yeah, and my sister, and the doctor, even had one of the nurses at the surgery talk to me.' She shook her head. 'But you don't tell me what I should be thinking or feeling, or doing.'

'I guess I don't.'

'Does my head in, you know, fed up with it.'

'Fed up?' Ian noted the interesting use of language but realised he might be attaching more meaning to it than was present for Mandy.

'People telling me what to do, what to think, on my case, you know?'

'Mhmm, I know what that can be like, but how is it for you?' Ian heard himself speak. The response sort of emerged from within him. It felt right though he wasn't sure how truly empathic it was. But then he recognised that in relationship thoughts, feelings and words could emerge that were timely and appropriate, particularly where there was some sense of connection present.

'I just feel like they're all trying to control my life.'

'Control your life?' Ian frowned slightly, curious as to what exactly Mandy was thinking and feeling as she said it.

'They never really bothered much in the past, let me sort of do my own thing, really, and now, now they just keep on at me – must eat, must put on some weight. For fuck's sake, can't they see I'm fat? Can't they see what's so bloody obvious?' Her voice had risen. Mandy was angry and irritated, and it showed.

'Really pisses you off that they can't see what you see.' Ian was aware of choosing his words carefully and wondered whether they would sound overly selective. He didn't want to collude with Mandy, as though he was taking sides with her, but then he didn't want her to feel he didn't believe what she was experiencing. The fact was, as he looked at her, there was no way that she was fat, and he quite understood why people were concerned, but that was not what Mandy was experiencing and if she wanted to explore this he had to accept her perception.

'Look at me. You think I'm fat?' Mandy looked at him, directly.

Ian knew he hadn't time to think, hesitation would not be helpful. He had to be honest with her, she wanted his view, maybe his view was important to her, or she was testing him in some way, he didn't know and he wasn't going to dwell on it. He responded, openly and honestly.

'Sitting here, looking at you, I don't see you as fat and I do accept and believe that your experience of yourself is that you are fat.' He wondered whether his response was too wordy, but it was what he felt, what he thought, what he saw. It felt like a moment of truth in their relationship. How would Mandy respond. He saw her staring at him, she didn't look too pleased.

This is a crucial moment. A direct question to which the counsellor responds, whilst also qualifying his response to try and convey an appreciation and an acceptance that his view is not his client's. It is a point to explore in supervision which the counsellor does.

'You're like everyone else, aren't you?'

'Is that how you experience me?'

'Hmm.' Mandy looked down. The truth was, no, it wasn't how she experienced him, but he was saying what they said, well, nearly. She took a deep breath and withdrew into her thoughts.

'It's not the response that you wanted to hear?' Ian was responding to the look on Mandy's face.

'It's what you think, isn't it?' Mandy shook her head, finding it hard to believe and yet, well, at the same time not exactly surprised either. Another adult telling her how it was. 'I thought I could trust you.'

'It feels to you like this is a matter of trust?'

Mandy nodded her head and looked away, taking a deep breath and sighing as she did so. 'I . . .' She didn't finish, what was the point? Why was she here? Why? Because her doctor wanted her to talk to someone, because her parents wanted her to eat more and put on weight. Put on weight! Couldn't they see she was already fat? She was shaking her head as she thought these things. And now, well, someone else.

For Ian he was aware of noting an urge within himself to try and patch up the relationship in some way, explain himself, but he also recognised that this was something he wanted. In fact, he needed to maintain his empathy for how Mandy was feeling and to continue to feel and communicate unconditional positive regard for her as the person she was, with all that was occurring for her as she sat there not wanting to hear what he had just said.

'I . . . ?' Ian wanted to maintain the thread of connection, it felt like a very fine thread all of a sudden and yet, somehow there was something quite intense as well about what was happening.

Mandy heard Ian's response. She still didn't know quite what to say. She felt let down, that was what it was, and back to feeling all alone, very much alone. No one seemed able, or willing, to see things the way she did, and she'd have to accept that, and she hated it, though she would push those feelings away when she could. It seemed like no one understood her, no one wanted to. She thought this counsellor would, did, but, well, what was the point.

Ian had noticed Mandy shaking her head. He decided to respond to this, not knowing what was the actual cause of this from within Mandy, but he didn't want to lose the connection with her, he didn't want her to feel like he was backing away from her, even if she wanted to back away from him, which she was perfectly entitled to do. But his job was to stay with her . . .

'Leaves you shaking your head, huh? Pissed off with me, yeah? It's a bugger hearing me say things that you don't want to hear.'

The counsellor empathises with what has occurred and in a sense offers a kind of empathic summary, with a certain quality of 'informed hunching' as to what the client may be feeling. He's reaching out, offering psychological contact. The counsellor is, in a sense, levelling with the client,

> seeking to say it as it is. He acknowledges the head movement, the feeling pissed off, and then seeks to convey an understanding of what he senses it must feel like.

Mandy sat, tight-lipped. Yeah, that summed it up, pretty much. She'd never quite had that response from anyone. But, well, that wasn't the point. He still thought she wasn't fat, not like she knew she was. How could he ... She shook her head again.

'You're like everyone else.'

'Because of my perception, I'm like everyone else?'

Mandy fidgeted in the chair, turning her body away from Ian. She didn't want to carry on with the counselling, waste of time, be better off just getting on with her life.

'Why did you have to say that?'

'I want to be honest with you. What's the point of me sitting here with you if I'm not being honest?'

'Huh.' Mandy heard the words but she wasn't impressed. 'Honest', she shook her head again and then stared down at the floor.

> The counsellor only needed to say the first part. The second part is unnecessary and is conveying criticism of his client. It may not be intentional. It may be a product of frustration. But it weakens the impact of the initial response.

'I'm going.'

'You want to go?'

Mandy said 'yes,' but at the same time could also feel something inside her saying, "no, stay", but she didn't know what that was about.

'OK, if that's what you honestly want to do, I don't want to stop you doing what you feel you need to do.'

'You mean I can go?'

'Sure, if that's what you want.'

'Oh, I don't know.' Mandy felt momentarily unsure, but she didn't know why. She just felt an urge to want to stay. And she didn't as well. She thought of the reactions of her parents, and her doctor, they'd all have a go at her. She was fed up with that and didn't want to go through all that hassle. Maybe she'd be better off staying, at least for a while, keep everyone happy. She didn't need them all in her face, at least being here, well, at least they thought she was doing something.

'I'll stay.'

'OK.' Ian smiled. He was genuinely pleased, aware of just how challenging it must have been for Mandy to hear him share his perception of her. He felt a warm acceptance for her, and whilst his smile was not a deliberate attempt to convey that, he felt sure that it was a product of that feeling.

'I don't want to change anything, though.'

'No, no, I'm sure you don't. Let everything be as it is, yes?'

'Yes ..., well, no, not everything, I mean, well, I just wish people would stop being mean to me.'

'Mhmm, that's what it's like, people being mean to you and you wish they'd stop.'

Mandy could feel herself breathing deeply and images of her parents' faces came into her mind's eye. And their voices, nagging at her, telling her to eat, telling her not to be so stupid, to do it for them even if she didn't want to do it for herself. What did they know? She was shaking her head again.

Ian noticed and commented. 'You shake your head a lot.'

'Hmm? Yeah, well, lots to shake it about. My parents, they don't understand. They seem to think there's something wrong, but, I mean, I'm fat, I can't seem to look like my mates. They all look so good, but me, I just can't stop putting on fat.' She shook her head. 'Not much point telling you, though, is it? You don't think I'm fat?'

'I don't see what you see, but I do believe and accept what you feel and experience.' Ian felt good as he spoke, he felt he was being genuinely honest, but not condemning her as wrong for what she experienced.

Does he need to explain himself again? Would a simple, 'no, I don't', have been sufficient? Or a 'no, I don't, but you do.' The wordiness of the counsellor's responses may be reflective of the fact that he is as much in his world as that of his client. It could be reflecting the fact that he finds it difficult to get into the inner world of his client, that perhaps it is, in some way, quite outside of his own experiencing. Maybe it is leaving him anxious, which he is not aware of, and this can also lead to unnecessary wordiness.

'How can you not see what I see? How can everyone else see ..., oh, what's the point.'

'Doesn't feel like there's much point talking about it?'

Mandy stared. She didn't shake her head. It was as though her frustration had taken her beyond that particular mannerism. What was there to say, do, to express how she felt. Utter frustration. And beneath that, though she wasn't experiencing it at the time, utter loneliness.

'What's wrong with everybody?'

'That's a question you'd really like answered and I guess I'm one of the "everybody"?'

'I'm not saying there's anything wrong with you,' Mandy felt herself flush a little, 'but you don't see me the way I do, do you?'

'It seems not.' He nodded slowly, taking a deep breath himself as he waited to see how Mandy would respond. He felt very focused and concentrated, aware that he needed to be fully present, heart and mind open and responsive to what Mandy was communicating.

'But I am fat.'

'Mhmm, you experience yourself as being fat.'

He could have responded, 'You feel fat.'

'But I am, I can't wear the sizes my friends get into.'

'Mhmm, and that makes you feel fat, not getting into the same sizes?'

'Yeah, course it does. But it's not just that, I mean, I'm fat, it makes me feel uncomfortable, I hate it, I hate my body, I hate being me.' Mandy's voice was raised by the time she had finished. She wasn't remembering, of course, that most of her friends were generally shorter than she was. Ian felt the anger, yet there was more than anger though he could not be sure exactly what. He stayed with the feeling he recognised.

'You hate your body, you hate being you, and you have so much anger about it.'

Mandy closed her eyes, she felt herself crumple inside. Yes, she was angry, but now, suddenly, now she felt very weak, very tired. She closed her eyes, they felt moist. Her heart was thumping. She didn't like what she was feeling. She stayed quiet, she felt so isolated, *no one* understood her, *no one* believed her. She rested her head against her right hand and continued to stare down at the carpet, seeing the colours in the fleck, but not really seeing them, not registering them. She sat, empty, no thoughts, just sat. She could feel her heart racing in her chest and her chest moving as she breathed in and out. Her hand was warm against the side of her face. She felt heavy, heavy ... She hated it. She continued to sit in silence, seemingly oblivious to where she was.

Ian was aware of feeling his own energy drain away, he also felt suddenly tired. It felt very present and he had learned to recognise that sometimes these intense experiences had relevance to the therapeutic process, even though he didn't really understand how they arose, or why.

'I don't know if this has meaning for you, but it all feels very tiring, as though all the energy drains away.'

Mandy felt herself slump down a little more. She could feel the waves of tiredness within herself and, yes, she just wanted to go to sleep and get away from everything and everyone, get away, disappear, be left alone. Just be left alone ....

'I'm so tired of it all, so tired.'

'Mhmm, so tired.'

Ian could feel himself wanting to yawn, he didn't stifle it. 'Gets to me, too,' he said after his yawn had finished. It triggered Mandy who yawned as well.

'Some days I don't have much energy.' Mandy had lifted her head and dropped her arm back down. It felt heavy. She felt like she was glued to the chair. She hated that feeling. Like a great big, fat, lump, that's how she felt.

'Mhmm, not much energy some days.'

'Gets me down, you know?'

'Gets you down not having much energy, feeling so tired.'

Mandy nodded. She'd never really talked quite like this before, and certainly not felt like someone was listening to her. She didn't know what to make of it. 'I wish I felt different, I wish I wasn't me.' She spoke with a sigh.

'That came from the heart, wishing you were different, wishing you weren't you.'

Mandy could feel herself going suddenly cold inside, and her arms felt strangely numb and yet sort of tingling at the same time. It was weird. She felt like her head was full of space and she felt suddenly distant, like she was disappearing into herself, like the walls of the room were becoming distant, she didn't like it. She blinked, and yawned again as another wave of tiredness hit her. She felt very weak.'

Ian saw the colour draining from Mandy's face. She had been quite pale anyway, but she seemed more pale all of a sudden.

'Mandy, are you OK?'

'I feel a bit strange.'

'Do you think you're going to faint?'

'I don't know.' She was now suddenly feeling like she was sweating, a kind of cold sweat.

'Do you want me to get the doctor, or the nurse? You might want to lie down.'

Mandy felt like she wanted to lie down, she didn't feel too good at all.

'I think I need to lie down.'

There wasn't a couch in the counselling room, Ian called reception. 'My client's feeling faint, she needs to lie down. Can one of the nurses or one of the doctors come in and is there a room with a couch that's free?'

There was, and there was soon a knock on the door.

'Come in.'

It was the practice nurse. 'Mandy's feeling very weak and wants to lie down, can we get her to one of the couches?'

'Sure, hello Mandy, come on, let's find somewhere for you to lie down.'

Mandy got slowly to her feet, and wobbled slightly as she found her balance. The nurse supported her and they went into the nursing room where there was a couch, and the nurse helped Mandy up on to it. 'I'm going to raise your feet, help the blood get back to your head, Mandy, OK.'

Mandy felt too weak to reply. But she mumbled 'OK'.

Ian stood by the couch, feeling concern. He'd never had a client suddenly feel faint like this before. Had he over-reacted? But he couldn't have let her lie on the floor in the counselling room. That didn't seem right.

The nurse's name was Annette. 'How are you feeling, Mandy?' She was taking her pulse.

Mandy swallowed, her throat felt very dry. 'Can I have some water?'

'I'll get some.' Ian went off to the water dispenser, returning a few moments later. 'Here you are.'

Mandy raised herself a little and sipped the water. She appreciated its coolness in her mouth and throat. She handed the plastic cup back to Ian and lay back down again. Her head was beginning to feel normal again.

'Do you often feel like this?'

'Sometimes, but not as bad as that. I mean, I feel tired sometimes, but that felt really weird.'

'Can you describe it?'

'Like I was sort of, I don't know, but I sort of felt small and weak and, I don't know, it's hard to describe.'

'Well, you just take it easy and don't rush to get up.'

Ian wasn't too sure whether to stay or head back into the counselling room. Annette was clearly going to stay and that felt right. He wasn't sure what impact a decision to leave might have, or even raising it. So he stayed. He glanced at his watch, the session would have been almost due to end, anyway. He knew he'd need to get himself ready for his next client in a few minutes. 'So, do you want to come back next week, same time, Mandy?'

Mandy lay on the couch looking at the lights in the ceiling and beginning to feel less light-headed. 'Yes, yes.' She smiled weakly. 'Thanks.'

'OK.'

'I'll stay with Mandy a little longer, you lie there till you feel ready to get up.'

The feeling faint occurred in a medical setting with other staff around. How might such a situation be handled in a different setting, if the client was being seen privately at the counsellor's home, for instance? The counsellor will want to reassure the client, but at what point might they feel they need to seek medical support? Also, in such a situation where you have a young girl and an older man, what implications does this have for the choices and decisions the counsellor might make? How does the gender mix affect the process? What issues might arise if there was a different gender mix/ age difference?

Ian said goodbye to Mandy and headed back into the counselling room. He wondered whether the fainting was simply physiological, or whether there was something psychosomatic in the experience. He knew how people could have unusual spacial experiences in therapy, particularly when encountering deep-seated feelings. Had that happened to Mandy, or was it that she was simply weak from not eating enough? Or both, of course? The truth was that he did not know, but he was glad she had agreed to come back the following week. And, well, she was in good hands now. He wondered whether the nurse would say anything about her eating, would she call the doctor? He didn't know. Was he right to call someone in? He felt he was. Mandy was clearly struggling and, well, he then wondered whether he should have trusted her process. But what if she had passed out, fell off the chair? No, he felt he had acted responsibly.

He wondered if he might have responded differently had he been a female therapist, and he guessed maybe he would, maybe he would have felt more at ease with allowing her to lie on the floor in the counselling room. But what was that about? Him? His gender? But would Mandy have felt OK about that? So many questions and he knew he needed to draw a line under that session and prepare himself for his next client. He decided to go outside for a breath of fresh air and take a cup of cool water out with him.

Points for discussion

- How has the session left you feeling and thinking? Explore what is present for you and reflect on how you would deal with it had you been Ian.
- What particular therapeutic strengths did you sense were present in the session?
- Evaluate the quality of Ian's empathy, congruence and unconditional positive regard.
- How might you have responded differently to Ian at any point in the session, and why?
- What would you take to supervision from this session?
- Write notes for this session.

CHAPTER 8

Counselling session 5: disclosures from the client's past

Ian had a little time before he was expecting Mandy to arrive and his thoughts drifted to a theme that had been with him a lot since that last session with her. It concerned the nature of trust and the role that it played in the person-centred counselling process. What did he trust, exactly? His client? But what did that mean? To behave in a certain way? No. That didn't feel right. People would be how they needed to be. He couldn't and shouldn't trust them to be a certain way. And yet trust was such an important feature, it seemed to him, of his attitude towards his client. So what was it?

The conclusion he had reached was one that he had read about (Rogers, 1986, p. 198) that: 'the person-centred approach is built on a basic trust in the person ... [It] depends on the actualizing tendency present in every living organism – the tendency to grow, to develop, to realize its full potential. This way of being trusts the constructive directional flow of the human being towards a more complex and complete development. It is this directional flow that we aim to release.'

He had found himself wanting to differentiate the person from the actualising tendency, and the psychology of the person from their behaviour. By offering the therapeutic conditions he felt he could trust the presence of the actualising tendency to bring about "constructive personality change". He felt warmly accepting of that notion. But this wasn't a trust in the person to be or to behave in a particular way. He had no idea what form of expression might flow out of that constructive personality change.

He thought of Mandy. The nurse had told him that she had headed off feeling much better, and that she had sought to encourage her to eat a little more, though Mandy hadn't really seemed very appreciative of being told that. No, thought Ian, that's not what she wants to hear at the moment. That, he thought, and the phrase seemed somewhat apt, is what she has had a belly-full of.

His thoughts went back to the actualising tendency. Yes, he trusted the presence of the actualising tendency in her – was it right to personalise it as *her* actualising tendency? Is it personal, he pondered, or an impersonal tendency that becomes personalised when it is present in a person ..., but if you take Rogers' idea of it being a kind of manifestation of a wider formative tendency ... What was it Rogers had written? Ian could remember a passage but had to work on remembering how it went. He took out a book from his bag and thumbed through it. Yes, there it was.

'I hypothesize that there is a formative directional tendency in the universe, which can be traced and observed in stellar space, in crystals, in micro-organisms, in more complex organic life, and in human beings. This is an evolutionary tendency toward greater order, greater complexity, greater inter-relatedness. In humankind, this tendency exhibits itself as the individual moves from a single-cell origin to complex organic functioning, to knowing and sensing below the level of consciousness, to a conscious awareness of the organism and the external world, to a transcendent awareness of the harmony and unity of the cosmic system, including humankind' (Rogers, 1980, p. 133).

"A process that gets disturbed and distorted by conditions of worth, by establishing beliefs about oneself that were rooted in other people's expectations, a process that gets disturbed on a macro-cosmic scale ..." He found himself thinking about ecology and the impact on nature of human-beings that showed little respect. He wondered ... what would happen if the therapeutic conditions were offered to nature, to the planet! Behaviour would change ... but what would it mean? He didn't know but somehow it felt important, that if this tendency found constructive expression in the person when certain conditions were present, would not the same be true at a collective level?

He brought his thoughts back to Mandy and her choice not to eat, and to maintain a view of herself that she was fat. Control. Trying to control bodily changes? He did not know for he did not yet know what Mandy experienced within herself to drive the perceptions that she had. He thought of the presence of the actualising tendency within her – was that the right way to describe it? Was it within her, or was it, in some sense best described as *being her*? Are we essentially a process of actualisation? He realised that his thoughts were beginning to make his head spin, and he smiled.

So much to ponder on, so much to grasp and make sense of. Yet in the therapy room it came down to a very simple reality. Did he, or did he not, trust in the presence of the actualising tendency? He knew that he did, not simply an intellectual knowing, it was a knowing that seemed to be present in his heart as well, and it felt to him that it was this that brought it alive. Yes, he thought, that is the essence of person-centred practice, that is the foundation, what it is built on. Bozarth is right, 'the foundation block of person-centred therapy is the actualizing tendency' (1998, p. 6). Unless you trust its presence and that the offering of the therapeutic conditions enables that tendency to operate towards "constructive personality change", you really cannot consider your-self to be client- or person-centred in your practice. It also brought to mind Bozarth's comment regarding the role of unconditional positive regard, 'in the context of person-centred theory, it is creating an atmosphere of unconditional positive regard that enables the person to develop unconditional positive self-regard and, subsequently, to resolve his or her specific problems' (1998, p. 5).

His thoughts returned again to Mandy. What was she feeling towards herself? What was driving her self-perception? It wasn't for him to try and find out, he knew the actualising tendency was present within her, as part of her, and that his unconditional positive regard would help her to begin to feel that uncondi-tional positive self-regard. He *knew it*. He smiled as he thought about how people so often, and so glibly, say "trust the process", and how shallow that often was. The process was deep, personal, human, took us to the limits, the depths, the essence of personhood. The actualising tendency *is* the process. Trust it.

He found himself taking a deep breath and glanced across at the clock. Five min-utes before Mandy was due to arrive. He decided to allow himself to be with his thoughts and to gently clear his mind ahead of the session, to help himself be open and sensitive to his experience of being with Mandy in the therapeutic relationship. He liked to do this before sessions. He would close his eyes and seek to be still. He knew it wasn't something everyone did, but it felt right for him.

When he opened his eyes it was almost time for the session to begin and he got up and went out to the waiting area. Mandy was sitting there, reading a magazine. As he approached, he saw it was a teenage publication and he guessed full of very thin girls conveying the image that the fashion industry wanted to por-tray. Or was he being prejudiced? He put the thought aside. 'Hello Mandy, good to see you, would you like to come through?'

She had looked up and put the magazine down in the table in the centre of the waiting room. 'Thanks.' She followed Ian to the counselling room.

Ian decided to ask if she was OK after last week. Yes, it was directing a focus, but it was an expression of his genuine concern for her well-being, and he recognised the therapeutic value in this.

It's a very warm and human thing to do. Sometimes it isn't only about what is communicated by what is said, but what is communicated by what goes unsaid. Unconditional positive regard is one of the therapeutic conditions, conveyed through warm acceptance of the client, of expressing normal human feelings of concern for the client's well-being. To not enquire might be seen as bringing the presence of unconditional positive regard into ques-tion. That would not be therapeutically helpful.

'You OK after last week?'

Mandy nodded. 'I felt weird, but I'm OK now.' Mandy thought of the way she had again been told that maybe she wasn't getting enough nourishment, that she should eat more. Always the same thing. Why couldn't people see that she was fat?

Ian nodded. He felt good that she was back. 'Well, I'm glad that you feel OK now.' He was genuine in what he said.

'Thanks.' Mandy looked away. She felt a little embarrassed. Her recollection had been that Ian had been so concerned. So had the nurse, but then she had started to talk to her about whether she was eating enough. Always the same. She felt mixed up inside. So many people on at her, and, well, they were all people she sort of didn't want to listen to, but Ian was sort of different. She couldn't explain it. Yes, she liked him, she knew that. Was it just that? She didn't know. What had he said before? Said he didn't see her as fat but respected how she saw herself. Well, she hadn't liked the first part, and still didn't, but no one else seemed to have at least tried to say they accepted how she saw herself. That *was* different. It still made her feel uncomfortable thinking about it. Was that the right word? She didn't know, sort of glad someone seemed to sort of want to accept her way, but clearly Ian also saw her the way everyone else did. She wanted to dismiss it, and in a way she did, and yet . . . it sort of kept nagging at her. Like it was unfinished in some way.

Ian sat and respected the silence that had developed between them. He thought of it that way. It wasn't that he was inwardly silent, and he imagined that it was the same for Mandy. It was just that nothing was being verbalised. But he could see from the concentrated look on Mandy's face that she was thinking about something. He had noticed her looking away. That moment had conveyed to him a sense of awkwardness or unease. What had he said? That he hoped she was feeling better, no, glad that she was feeling OK. How had she received that? He didn't know, but maybe some part of her was attaching a meaning to his words that was causing something to be experienced in Mandy. He let his thoughts go. He wasn't there to be sidetracked into his own internal speculations although he acknowledged that it happened. He focused back on Mandy. She was still looking away. It seemed to him that she had a frown on her face.

'You look very concentrated, but I don't want to disturb your train of thought.'

Mandy felt awkward, unsure of herself. She didn't know what to say. People in her head, telling her what was good for her. She didn't want to listen to them. Just wanted to escape, yes, escape inside herself . . . , and yet she didn't feel comfortable inside herself either. It was hard to think about, more a kind of feeling, a sensation. She felt troubled but she didn't know what by. She knew what she knew about herself; it was everyone else who didn't understand, who just wanted to tell her how to be. She'd had that at home so much. She didn't know how she wanted to be, and it felt scary, frightening. She didn't know . . . Her heart was beating, well, pounding, in her chest and she felt herself take a deep breath. She didn't like feeling like this. She just felt like she had no control over her life, except what she chose to eat and not eat. At least she had that.

She wanted to talk about it, about ''things'' but she didn't know who to talk to. It wasn't something she talked about to her friends, everyone was too busy having a good time. Her parents, well, they'd go on about her not eating properly. Her brother? No, wasn't something she felt she could talk to him about, and her sister, well, they'd never really been that close. Truth was she felt quite alone, at least inside herself. And here she was with a counsellor, someone who you were supposed to talk to but she couldn't. She shook her head slightly. It felt uncomfortable sitting, not saying anything. Her heart was still thumping in her chest and her throat, she realised, had gone quite dry. She felt a little "spaced out", and on edge. She didn't like it.

Ian wanted to acknowledge again that he was there, willing to listen but also prepared to respect his client's silence. 'I don't know what is happening for you, Mandy, and I know it's not always easy to talk, but if you want to I'd really like to hear what you have to say.'

When breaking a silence it is important for the counsellor to be clear as to their motivation. Who are they doing this for? Is it to ease their own sense of disconnection? Is it to convey their presence as a therapeutic response? Is it something else? Counsellors can learn a great deal about themselves when they honestly and openly reflect on what becomes present for them during a silence.

Mandy felt tears in her eyes. She suddenly felt quite sad and wasn't sure why. Not that she thought about it, it was suddenly there. She closed her eyes and felt a tear trickle down her cheek. She swallowed, she wanted to say something, but she didn't know what. It felt like there was a pressure inside herself to speak, say something, anything, release the tension inside her. 'I don't know what to say.'

Ian noted Mandy's expression and had also noted the tear. 'Don't know what to say. Sadness?'

Mandy nodded. She hadn't felt sad when she had arrived for the counselling, but she did now. Sad, suddenly frightened as well, but she didn't know what of. She knew there were things she didn't like about herself, but she just felt unhappy and she didn't really know why. Her thoughts turned to her granny who had died two years ago. She used to talk to her. Somehow, well, somehow she was different. She did listen. She did somehow seem to . . . , she didn't know how to describe it, but she was just there in a different kind of way. She missed her. Yes, it had been bad enough facing the future when she was there, but now, well, now she felt so alone with it. She spent time with her friends, but somehow she felt different. Set apart somehow. She couldn't explain it.

'I miss my Gran.'

'Your Gran was special?'

Mandy nodded, and felt tears in her eyes. She swallowed and reached for a tissue. 'She was someone I could sort of talk to, you know?'

Ian nodded, 'yeah, someone to talk to'. Ian was aware that Mandy had not mentioned her Gran before. His immediate thought was that she had maybe died, but he wasn't going to express his thoughts. That was not relevant. He needed to maintain the therapeutic attitude and allow Mandy to explore further if she wished.

Mandy was sighing. 'She, I don't know, she listened. She, I don't know, things were different with her. Not so chaotic. I mean, at home it's chaotic, you know, sort of do your own thing really, which is great, but ... I used to like seeing Gran. She was so organised. I mean, I don't know, it was different.'

'Hard to describe, something about being organised, but it was certainly different for you when you were with her.'

'She died, though, nearly two years ago now.' She shook her head as she stared down at the floor. 'So much I wanted to say to her. Makes me feel sad thinking about her.'

'Missing her, missing not being able to talk to her, tell her the things you want to tell her. That's sad.'

Mandy heard Ian's voice and what he was saying was just so true. She was thinking back to the times when they had talked, she'd been worried about, well, maturing as a woman. She wasn't sure about her body, what was happening to her. Her mother never really seemed to understand. Told her to not worry, that it was how it was. But for Mandy it was everything. Her body was changing. The way she felt was changing. She saw how women looked in the magazine and she, well, she didn't feel like them. She didn't feel like she would stay slim like they were. She'd talk to her Gran about it, and she'd listen and reassure her. And that sort of helped, somehow, but when she had gone, well, then she had no one to talk to about it, not how she really felt. She'd tried talking to friends but they somehow didn't see it the way she did.

Mandy stayed silent, she didn't know what to say. She felt so much inside herself and it sort of filled her, gave her no room to say anything. Strange feeling, but it was like everything was happening on the inside and, well, it felt hard to say anything. She sniffed and blew her nose on a tissue.

Ian sat with his attention on Mandy. He felt pleased that she had disclosed about her Gran. She was obviously a key figure in Mandy's life. He wanted to be sure that he conveyed his warm acceptance to Mandy for what she was feeling. Her Gran dying two years ago – Mandy would have been 15 – a time of change for her and a lot to cope with. He felt for her.

'I wish she was still here. Things would be different. I sometimes think about what she might say, but, well, it's sort of faded. It's like I don't know what she'd say now, except, "come on dear, cheer up, it's never as bad as you think". She often said that. I want to think it's true, but I don't know. I just don't know what I want, it's like, I just don't want to ..., I don't know, anything.'

'Don't want to "anything"?'

'What's the point. I miss her.'

'Yeah, you really miss her.'

Mandy nodded. She looked up at Ian. 'What do I do?'

'About?'

'Everything. I mean, I just feel so alone, I just don't want to ...,' Mandy didn't finish the sentence though the words formed in her head. They summed up her fears, her dilemma, but they seemed hard to say, somehow. They sort of were in her head and that's where they stayed.

'Something you don't want to . . . ?' Ian's empathic response was in the form of a question, inviting Mandy to say more. He didn't want to push her. He could sense the sensitivity around what was being explored. He recognised that, for whatever reason, Mandy was struggling to voice something, or maybe she simply didn't want to. Again, he knew his role was to maintain the therapeutic attitude and provide that relational experience for Mandy to be as she needed to be, as she wanted to be, as she was able to be, without his presence in any way imposing direction or conditioning upon her.

The counsellor seeks to be facilitative, conveying that he has heard Mandy say something and then stop, offering opportunity for her to say more if she wishes. A questioning empathic response is not something offered with deliberate intent to cause something to happen. If it was, that would argu-ably be directive and not strictly person-centred practice. The counsellor can usefully ask themselves: am I asking in order to enable the client to say more if they wish, am I asking in order to make the client say something, or am I asking to clarify my own understanding of what is happening for my client? The case above is, perhaps, tending more towards the first motivation to enquire. The second motivation would clearly not be person-centred.

Mandy thought about what was in her head. She hadn't realised it but she was rubbing her hands together, holding her fingers tightly as she rubbed them. Ian noted the hand movements and sensed the tension that was present. He didn't say anything, he didn't want to take Mandy's attention away from what was happening for her. 'Not easy to talk about . . .'

Mandy nodded, yet somehow she knew she had to. Who else was there to talk to? She felt that maybe she could trust Ian, at least he seemed to listen. Yes, he'd made her feel pissed off when he'd said how she looked to him in the last ses-sion. And that still niggled at her. But this was different, this was something else, this was nothing to do with that – at least, that was how she saw it. She took a deep breath.

'I just feel like I don't want to grow up.' She'd said it. It sort of felt a relief and yet she felt suddenly anxious as well, wondering what Ian would say. It sort of sounded stupid now she'd said it, and yet she knew it wasn't, she knew that was what she felt.

'Don't want to grow up, doesn't feel good.' Ian spoke softly.

Mandy shook her head. 'I don't know what I want, I really don't. I mean, I wish I could go back to how things were.'

'How things were?'

'When Gran was alive, I mean, everything seemed so easy then. Didn't have to worry about things like I do now. So much to have to think about, growing up, exams, jobs, boys, becoming a woman, so much going on.'

'So much going on in your life.'

'And it goes round and round inside me.'

'Yeah, feels like it's all inside you, going round and round.'

'Like I can't control it, can't control anything. I hate it.' Mandy felt the sadness arising, and the anxiety, the fear, the feeling that everything was out of control, everything. She began to cry.

'You hate not feeling in control, yeah, it's so upsetting, so hard to cope with.'

Mandy nodded through her tears. She reached over for another tissue. 'Gran would know what to do, but she's not here.' Another wave of sadness, of grief, more tears. Mandy sat looking down holding the tissue to her face, sobbing.

Ian felt his heart go out to the girl, young woman before him. She was a young woman and yet she was so much a little girl overwhelmed by experience, by being on that inevitable journey into adulthood, so scared, so frightened, so wishing things could be like they were when she was a child and her Gran was alive.

'She'd know what to do.'

Mandy heard Ian's response. Yes, she thought, Gran would know what to do.

For Ian, he could see how Mandy's not eating was linked but he was not going to start making connection into that part of Mandy's life. That was for Mandy to make. For now, he would continue to provide the therapeutic climate to enable Mandy to openly be herself, express herself and maybe, as a result of feeling heard, accepted, validated in her feelings, begin to find her own way forward. And maybe, in that process, she might gain a fresh perspective on herself, her eating, her size. But he wasn't going to say anything. It could simply block the process and, anyway, would not be expressive of a person-centred way of working. He trusted the presence of the actualising tendency. Mandy had found a way to try and cope with feeling out of control. She controlled her eating, her body as best she could. She would only stop this if and when she felt she was gaining control in other parts of her life. That was his belief.

Mandy had begun to speak again. 'She just, I don't know, she'd calm me down, if I got worried. She'd say how things would be OK, that she'd worried like I did, do. But there are so many more things to worry about. I mean, I'd only started to think about, you know, growing up and stuff back then. And then she got ill and was in hospital, and that was horrible to see. She just suddenly became so old.' Mandy shook her head, memories clearly in her mind, and the tears once again very present in her eyes. Her throat burned and felt raw. She took a sip of water from the polystyrene cup beside her. It felt cool, but it did nothing to ease the pressure in her head and the churning feeling in her stomach.

Ian nodded, 'so distressing to see her become old like that. Horrible for you to see.'

Mandy nodded slightly herself. She was back in the hospital. She could see her Gran lying there. She seemed so small, so frail, so grey. Her hair all wispy. Her eyes had begun to look dull. She didn't understand. Now, well, she guessed it might have been the medication, though she didn't know. But it was like she wasn't her Gran any more, and yet she was. But she wasn't, not the Gran who laughed and played with her and gave her hugs and home-made cake, and told her not to worry, everything would be alright. How she'd say 'look at me, life's good, it'll be good for you, too'. But it hadn't been good. She'd changed, she became someone else. She did look at her. Life was not good and it wouldn't be good for her.

'I don't want to get old.'

'You don't want to get old because of what you saw then?'

Mandy nodded. 'I don't want to, I don't know, I just . . . , I don't know.'

'You just don't know, yeah?'

Mandy nodded. She looked across at Ian. He seemed to be so concerned, somehow. She forced a smile through tight lips, and felt her lower lip begin to tremble as another wave of emotion swept through her and her eyes filled with tears once again. 'I-I'm s-sorry.'

'No need to be sorry. So much you feel sad and worried about. Let it out if you want to.'

The tears continued to flow. 'I miss her so much. There's no one like her, how she was, no one.'

'Yeah, no one quite like your Gran. She was one of a kind, huh?'

A very human touch to this response. It adds to the power. This is not given with the intention of it being this way, it is a natural, human response and it conveys something to the client.

Mandy felt herself smile and as she did so more tears welled up in her eyes. 'Yeah, yeah, she was, she really was.' Somehow hearing Ian say that somehow sort of made a difference, somehow. 'Yes, she was one of a kind.' Her Gran. *Her* Gran. She remembered suddenly playing ball in the garden with her, how her Gran was always hitting it over the fence, and then having to go around and ask for the ball back. She felt like a friend, somehow, yes, a friend. A special friend. A really special friend.

Mandy looked up again. 'And I've got to get on without her, haven't I?'

'You have her memory, but yes, life has to go on now without her.'

Mandy was nodding to herself. Yes, she knew that, but it was so scary. She felt so . . . , she couldn't put it into words to herself, let alone to Ian. 'It's like, I don't know.'

'Like you don't know?'

'Like I don't know, I mean, what to do, what I want to do, I just don't know.'

'Don't know what you want to do?'

'Everyone else seems to, and, I mean, I guess I'll do what I need to do, go to university, that's what my mum and dad want. And I should, I mean, I know they're right. But . . .' she sighed, 'what for? I don't know what I want to do. So many things to have to think about and decide. I don't know. Gran used to encourage me, told me it was important that I do well. She used to say that . . .' Mandy went quiet as a memory surfaced. It made her feel strangely numb.

'She used to say ...?' Ian spoke gently, not wanting his response to be experienced as pressurising. He just wanted to gently acknowledge what Mandy was saying and acknowledge that he had heard her not finish her sentence.

'She'd say that childhood could be the best time of your life – enjoy it. I did, with her, and with friends, but now, well, now I wonder, if this is as good as it gets, I mean, people do say that about childhood, don't they, happiest days of your life.'

'They do say it. And it's something that's clearly meant something for you.'

'Does It get better?'

'It can do. It certainly gets different.' Ian smiled, he wanted to offer some kind of reassurance yet at the same time he also wanted to convey a warm acceptance of what Mandy was experiencing and feeling. 'It seems like you're not so sure, and that gives you feelings ...'

Mandy nodded. 'I'd like to think it can be better, and I suppose it can. I just can't see it. I mean, so much to think about, worry about, you know? So much ...'

'Yeah, being an adult can mean lots to think about.'

Mandy shook her head. 'I just wish ..., I don't know, I know I can't go back. I mean, I'd like to but I know I can't, not really.' She rubbed her eyes, they were beginning to itch.

'Yeah, you'd like to go back to how it was, back when your Gran was alive, but, yeah, you know you can't.'

'And, I've got to think more positively, haven't I, about the future, even though I don't want to think about it.'

'That sounds like you don't want to but there is a pressure that you should.'

Mandy nodded. 'Mum and Dad, how many times have they told me to "grow up". Just makes me not want to even more.'

'Parents, huh, telling you what's right for you.'

'And I guess they're right. That's what's such a pain, you know?'

Ian nodded. 'Mhmm. Can be hard to accept your parents are right sometimes.'

'Yeah.'

Ian had noticed the time, the session was due to end in a few minutes. 'We've only got a few more minutes left, and you've really worked hard today. I want to acknowledge that, and say I appreciate how you've talked about your Gran, and how you feel about her, about the past and the future. None of it is easy.' Ian felt strongly he wanted to acknowledge all of this, make his experience visible to his client. She had worked hard, it had been a very emotional session. How Mandy would be affected, he didn't know. But she had connected with feelings and, he hoped, felt them validated by his acceptance of her, of them, of how she needed to be.

'No, no, it isn't, but I think I needed to talk about these things. Actually it wasn't as hard as I thought, I mean it was, but once I started telling you things, well, it was OK.'

'You feel OK to head off, or is there anything else for today?'

'No, I need to head off – homework to do.'

Ian nodded and smiled. 'Yeah, there's always homework.'

Mandy nodded.

'Same time next week, OK?'

Mandy nodded again. 'Thanks, yes, I'm glad I came. Did wonder about it, but, well, thanks.' She got up. Ian watched her leave before turning to sit back in his chair and reflect on the session.

Points for discussion

- If you were the counsellor at the end of the session, what would be the focus of your reflections?
- Evaluate the way in which the counsellor continued to create a therapeutic relationship in this session.
- What were the key moments? Identify two particularly significant responses from Ian, and explain why they proved therapeutically helpful.
- What would you take to supervision from this session?
- Write notes for this session.

CHAPTER 9

Supervision: processing the response to a direct question

Ian had been working with Nina for a year and their supervisory relationship had developed into one of mutual respect. Nina saw Ian once a month and Ian would use the time to explore issues that had arisen in relation to his client work, although sometimes the sessions took on a more theoretical focus though generally as a result of something that had occurred in a counselling session. They had also focused on the supervisory relationship itself, and explored what was said and what may be left unsaid, what did Ian bring to supervision and what did he leave out, and why. They had realised that the focus was often more on problems and difficulties and Nina had been keen to ensure that there was also time to acknowledge achievements and a sense of "good practice" as well.

'I know I've mentioned Mandy before, the girl who is very underweight and has been sent to me for counselling.'

Nina nodded, 'yes, though she really hasn't wanted to say much about it.'

'That's right. Well, it's been interesting.'

'Interesting.' Nina couldn't resist the smile. She loved it when a supervisee said that something was interesting. It was one of those words that never really conveyed what was to follow.

Ian smiled. He knew he was in the habit of over-using that word. 'OK, well, let's be more specific, though it has been interesting as well . . .'

'OK.'

'Mandy asked me a direct question a couple of sessions back about how I saw her.'

'In what sense?'

'Physically, her size. I forget exactly how it came up, but it was a direct question and it was one of those moments when you know it demands a direct answer, not a "it seems important for you to know what I think", you know?'

'Mhmm, I do. What made it feel that way, though? How did you discern that, what sounds like, a kind of demand from Mandy?'

'The look on her face, the way she spoke. It was like, "OK, level with me, let's get real here".'

'And you did?'

'Well, I said what I thought, that she didn't look fat to me but that I accepted that wasn't how she saw, experienced, herself.'

'In that order?'

Ian smiled. 'Good point. Yes, yes, it was in that order. Yes, I gave my experience of her first and then said about accepting her view. You think I should have said it the other way around?'

Nina shrugged. 'I don't know about should, it's something that struck me.'

Ian frowned as he thought about it. 'OK, let me say it the other way, see what it sounds like. "I really accept how you see yourself Mandy, I really do, and I know that it isn't how I see you. I don't see you as being fat." Something like that?'

'How does it feel to you?'

'More accepting of her view and less centred on mine . . .' Ian paused. 'But then she did ask for my view. The question was, as I recall, "do you think I'm fat?". That was the question to which I said, well, I said "no" to, but then qualified it.'

'Mhmm. I just think it's interesting to consider the contrast.'

'It is. And I am wondering how Mandy would have felt. She might have thought I was hedging if I'd qualified it first. It just felt like a direct question demanding a direct answer.'

'Yes, and I am sure you are right. You were in relationship in the moment that the question was asked.'

'And you're right as well to open it up. It's an interesting one. I don't know if she'd have responded differently. She told me I was like everyone else.'

'Everyone else . . . ?'

'Telling her she needed to put on weight.' Ian paused. 'I didn't go as far as that, but I guess that's how she may well have heard it. She said something about trust, not being able to trust me – I guess because of my not seeing what she sees.'

Nina nodded and was aware of feeling a sense of what an important question that Mandy asked, and wondering how she might have responded, or felt, had she been Ian. 'I'm just wondering how I might have felt had I been faced with that question. It really is a huge moment, isn't it?'

Ian nodded. 'And I knew I had to be honest, not hesitate, simply say what I felt. And, well, I didn't know whether the relationship would take it, you know? She could have marched out of the door, could have, but didn't. I guess she was left with a sense of not trusting me to see what she saw, but how she then interpreted that, I don't know.'

'How do you mean?'

'Well, I didn't say what Mandy wanted to hear, or at least what the part of her that sees her as fat wanted to hear. Maybe there's another part of her that thinks differently, but that's not been made visible to me, not yet, anyway.'

'That's interesting, you mean like a kind of configuration within her sense of self?'

'Yes, so, I mean, I could say that I was speaking to that part, but, well, I wasn't, I certainly had no intention like that, and wouldn't want to, actually. I wanted to simply respond to Mandy in the moment. I'm not interested in . . . , well, it's

OK to reflect on it theoretically, but at the time, well, you can end up playing games if you start thinking about talking to different parts of the person, particularly the parts that aren't speaking.'

'And that may not even exist!'

'Quite. So, in the session I responded to my experience of Mandy, there, in front of me, wanting to know whether I saw her as fat.'

'Mhmm.'

'But this question of trust and how she experienced my response. Yes, she couldn't then trust me. I guess, to see things how she experienced them. OK. But what she did with that, I don't know. I mean, she could have decided well, "can I trust him at all because he is telling me something that is plainly wrong because I know I am fat". And it would be reasonable to then feel she couldn't trust me. Why should she?'

'Why should she trust you?'

'Then again, she might have felt, well, he's wrong, but at least he's being honest, and he is saying he believes me in what I'm feeling and experiencing – but then, I don't know, that might feel patronising, you know, sort of "there, there, I know you see you like that, but I see you like this". It's messy, isn't it?'

Nina nodded. 'So many possibilities here.'

'I could have just said, "no, I don't see you as fat". And, well, maybe that would have been more, I don't know – helpful? But would it? I wanted her to feel heard in terms of how she sees herself.'

'Only heard?'

'Validated? I mean, . . . , hmm, I'm also aware that we hadn't maybe really formed a therapeutic relationship – maybe I was trying too hard to achieve that, using it as an opportunity to sort of get alongside, as it were, and say "hey, I'm not like everyone else, not really. What I've just said might sound like everyone else, but, you know, I at least accept how you see yourself"'.'

'So you think you may have used that moment to try and establish a clearer therapeutic connection?'

'That doesn't feel right?'

'Doesn't feel right?'

'More doesn't feel appropriate.'

'OK, doesn't feel appropriate to use the moment in that way.'

'No, certainly not intentionally. I mean, my role is to be congruent, to be integrated into the relationship, experience and convey unconditional positive regard and to communicate my empathic understanding of what my client is telling me or experiencing.'

'OK, agreed, we don't think, "aha, here's a moment to establish therapeutic relationship".'

'But should I have just given the direct answer without the qualification? And yet I was being genuine in what I said. I think if I had a sense at the time of saying it for a reason other than because that was what I was experiencing, then it would be questionable. I don't feel I was doing that, but I can't rule out that maybe somewhere inside me there was an urge to do this.' Ian blew out a breath. 'And yet, what's interesting is that Mandy has come back and in the last session there was much more disclosure from her about her past, although I don't recall much, if anything, being said about her eating pattern. So it feels like there is a trust, she has trusted me with some parts of herself, but not the parts specific to the eating, well, even saying that, what she said in the last session has to be linked, but she's not making the link or at least not communicating it to me.'

'OK, so she's still engaging in the relationship and your sense is that she feels sufficiently trusting of you to make certain other disclosures ...'

'... quite painful ones.'

'Quite painful disclosures.'

'She talked about her Gran, how important she was in her childhood. Her Gran died I think she said two years ago – Mandy would have been about 15. Her Gran was someone she could talk to, and someone who reassured her. She sounds like a much more steady influence than her parents.'

'Mhmm, stability, and a really important person.'

'I think not having her Gran to talk to has had a major impact on Mandy, and I wonder how it will have left her feeling, talking about her Gran to me, and how it feels not having her around. It feels like a really important area for her to have talked about. I remember saying something about how her Gran sounded like one of a kind, something like that. I don't know, something felt sort of different in that moment, somehow, like I was now offering reassurance for what Mandy experienced. I hadn't thought of it quite like that until now, but maybe, in a strange way, maybe I've sort of ... Hmm, it's not that I can replace her Gran, but maybe I can offer the stability that she lost when her Gran died?'

'Mhmm.'

'Which then, well, I mean, I know some schools of thought would be thinking about projection or transference and I know I don't think that way, rather I will seek to be congruently myself and convey warm acceptance of how Mandy needs to be.'

'You will be Ian the counsellor.'

Ian nodded. 'I may convey something that for Mandy has echoes or resonance, as it were, with her experience of being with her Gran, but I am not her. But I can offer her a place to come and talk and, well, maybe in time she may then begin to trust me – or maybe trust herself – to explore other areas. I mean, she's already talked about how life feels out of control, she's afraid of growing up, doesn't know what to do. Oh, and seeing her Gran dying in hospital, seeing how people can become, that also made a big impression as well. I think she's just feeling overwhelmed with so much, and during a period in her life when she lost the one person she had learned to turn to and trust.'

'It sounds like Mandy has moved on.'

'She is being more present – no, I mean, she was present but more silently present. She's more visibly expressive now, she's moved, shifted. She's being, expressing feelings in the session, within the therapeutic relationship. Yes, towards a particular set of experiences, but, well, people don't reveal everything about everything at the same time.' Ian was thinking of Rogers' seven stages, that how perhaps different parts of the person might be at different stages. Clearly Mandy was exhibiting feelings towards her Gran in the session, in the relationship. But feeling, thoughts, experiences towards her body, shape, size, eating were not being communicated.

'No, bit by bit, as they feel able and ready.'

'Trusting the presence of the actualising tendency, knowing that, as the theory suggests, if the relational climate is present, constructive personality change can occur. And clients will bring those aspects or parts of themselves that they feel ready and able to bring into that therapeutic experience.'

'And we trust the timeliness of that process – at least, we do if we are genuinely person- or client-centred in our practice.'

Ian nodded. 'Yes, so for me it is about maintaining my therapeutic attitude, encouraging the presence of the therapeutic climate and allowing Mandy to bring of her herself what she does, trusting the presence of the actualising tendency.'

'Trusting its existence and trusting that her internal process will make best use of what you are offering.'

'And that's the challenge, particularly in an instance like this. I mean, hypothetically, what if the client's eating pattern – let's say her anorexic condition – was putting her life at risk.'

'How do you mean?'

'Well, I'd want to communicate my acceptance of her need to be that way, yes?'

'Mhmm.'

'And I might express my feelings as well, as a human-being with someone who was following a course of action that could lead to her death.'

'Yes, transparency.'

'And I'd want to convey my unconditional positive regard, I mean, you know, unconditional, that my positive regard is not conditional on her eating, or not. And that seems to be what is so crucial, to convey that warmth, that caring, that heartfelt whatever it is because I'm a human-being and am affected by another person's choice.' Ian paused. 'It's love, isn't it? I know it's simplistic to say that people who don't feel love for themselves – from others and from themselves – but that's the big barrier to . . .' Ian paused, uncertain of what words to use.

'Big barrier to . . . ?'

'People, I don't know, finding fulfilment, creating a satisfying lifestyle, being accepting of themselves, yes, something about, now, what was it, yes, I remember reading about positive self-regard. Yes, how that's key, enabling people to experience positive self-regard and that's what we are offering clients the opportunity to develop and experience.'

The possibility of experiencing unconditional positive self-regard is encouraged by the experience of receiving unconditional positive regard. Can I accept myself as I am? Can I? Or am I beset by conditions of worth that are rooted in either conditional regard which may have been positive or negative? The person-centred counsellor accepts that by offering the therapeutic conditions that the likelihood is that the client will begin to experience some degree of unconditional positive self-regard. It may be small, and may take time to become established, particularly for a client with deep-seated 'conditions of worth', but it is an important stage in the process of the client reorganising their internal attitude and relationships within and with themselves.

'So by offering the therapeutic conditions, that is a key factor, a key result area, the fostering of positive self-regard in the client.'

'And yes, I can accept that someone may need medical "treatment" to keep them alive, that's a different order of intervention. But then there has to be an opportunity given for the client to explore whether they might feel different towards themselves. I think that's an important part of what we offer clients. So, an anorexic client that physiologically needs a medical intervention is, perhaps, in a sense buying time for therapeutic relationship to create the relational climate for the actualising tendency to foster positive self-regard, something like that.' Ian paused, aware of feeling quite thoughtful. 'There's a lot to ponder on in all of this, but it goes to the core of what the person-centred approach offers to people. We simply trust our clients and that trust seems intimately linked to the notion of an actualising tendency and of the role of the necessary and sufficient conditions in encouraging the possibility of constructive personality change. And there are no guarantees of any particular change occurring, or how much, and where there is a specific behaviour concerned whether the "constructive psychological change" will be of a nature such that it might change the behaviour.' Ian paused again, 'and yet whatever the approach there is never any guarantee, but it feels like there is an honesty and an integrity in the person-centred approach in the way that we own the fact of uncertainty around behaviour change. Yes, we offer a therapeutic relationship that we know can, and does, foster constructive personality change. It is then whether this will then in turn foster "constructive behaviour change" – and then we have the problem of who defines what this means for a particular person in the context of their own experience.'

'Other approaches see constructive behaviour change as a goal, and have a specific behaviour change in mind to aim for, believing that this is what the client needs, or is best for them, or whatever. But, yes, we believe that the actualising tendency will foster constructive personality change in the context of a therapeutic relational experience as defined by Rogers. And we believe that, well, I believe, that for constructive behaviour change of any kind to be sustainable and meaningful to the person themselves it has to be underpinned and informed by constructive personality change.'

Ian nodded. 'So, back to Mandy, she will change her eating behaviour – labelled anorexic within the medical model – in a truly sustainable way when she changes internally in a manner that leaves her no longer needing the behaviour.'

'Yes. And whilst that change has not occurred then she is likely to need that behaviour and is likely to continue with it and, if she is forced into change, will be at risk of relapsing back into her anorexic pattern.'

'Sustainable change – that's what it's about, isn't it?'

'It always is, isn't it?'

Ian nodded. He suddenly felt quite enlivened by the discussion, and felt somehow more positive towards Mandy and what he was offering her. Yes, he thought, yes, it reinforced his own awareness of the importance of what he offered to the relationship. Accept her as she is, don't push her, feel and communicate unconditional positive regard, be open and genuine, be a companion but don't direct, and listen so that she feels heard and more freely able to be herself and move around within herself.

The session drew to a close and Ian left feeling refreshed and renewed. It felt an important session, enabling him to in a sense reconnect with first principles.

Points for discussion

- How helpful do you feel this supervision session was in enabling Ian to prepare himself for his next session with his client?
- Would it have satisfied you, as the counsellor?
- What do you think about the link between 'constructive personality change' and 'constructive behaviour change'?
- As a supervisee, what would you take from this supervision session?
- Write notes for this session as the supervisee.

CHAPTER 10

Counselling session 6: the internal world begins to break down

Ian was looking forward to the next session with Mandy. That previous supervision session, he realised, had helped him to clarify his own thinking, particularly around the links between "personality change" and "behaviour change". He had pondered on that theme a lot after the supervision and felt much more secure in his role of offering a relational climate that primarily was concerned with "constructive personality change" and feeling able to trust that behaviour change that may flow would be expressive of it and would take the form that the client found most fulfilling or satisfying.

He glanced at the clock, Mandy was due to arrive. He went out and found her waiting and called her. When Mandy had sat down, Ian asked her how she wished to use the time they had.

Mandy had had a strange week. She had felt strangely close to her Gran, so many memories had flooded back, things she knew but somehow they were suddenly more present in a strange kind of way. She could see herself with her Gran and yet there was one aspect of her memories that troubled her, and she was uncertain what to do about it. And she didn't really feel she wanted to talk about it given what Ian had said in that earlier session. But she felt she could say a bit about the memories. 'Been thinking about Gran a lot.'

'Mhmm.'

Mandy had actually got some photos out one evening, pictures of her Gran, and of her with her. She'd looked at those pictures and they somehow seemed to be of another time, almost of another person. She knew it was her in the pictures with her Gran, and yet . . . , somehow she seemed like someone else. It had felt uncomfortable. Here was the little girl that she had been, that she still wanted to be, and yet somehow she was so different, so distant, so . . . , so . . . , other. She didn't really know how to describe it, or whether she wanted to.

'Last week left you thinking about her a lot . . .' Ian felt he wanted to acknowledge what Mandy had said. Somehow, on reflection, "mhmm" didn't seem enough.

> The counsellor is right. What Mandy had said was important to her. The counsellor knows that her Gran means a lot to her. 'Mhmm' does not acknowledge enough, however it might be said. Sometimes the counsellor needs to use more words to convey more than the words. That may sound strange, but communicating empathic understanding, unconditional positive regard and congruence may need enough words in order to express oneself through a tone of voice. There is only so much tonal expression that can be conveyed through 'mhmm'.

Mandy nodded. 'It's funny. I mean it was sort of upsetting, but not really, not like it was when I was here. I can't explain it.'

'Sort of upsetting but not exactly, and not as much as it was when you were here last week. Something like that?

Mandy nodded. 'I don't know. Just think about her a lot, thinking about what she'd say to me now, and what I'd say to her.'

'Like having conversations with her, what would you say, what would she say.' Ian nodded slightly himself and smiled slightly. Somehow it seemed like a really important thing for Mandy to have been doing and as far as he was concerned had a very touching feel to it.

'And I know she'd reassure me, you know? Probably tell me how it would be OK. Never thought she'd die, I mean, you don't do you? Thought she'd always be there for me, forever and ever.'

Ian felt goosebumps breaking out. Was it a memory of his own from childhood that was being touched? He didn't know. But, yes, you didn't think people like your Gran would die, not when you were a young child, anyway.

'Yeah, forever and ever.' He knew the way he spoke was expressing something of his own reaction.

'She is, in my head, but that's not enough. I need her to talk to.'

'Need her to talk to, things you want to say to her?'

> The counsellor has strayed from the client's frame of reference. He only needed to confirm that he had heard her need to talk to her. He has, potentially, shifted the focus from the 'need' to the 'thing' that she might want to say. It may seem small, but it is a shift of emphasis and could be viewed as directive and therefore not person-centred. Being a person-centred counsellor or therapist is a discipline. It is a challenge. Those who think being person-centred is a soft-option, or an easier way to be a therapist are mistaken.

'And it's about her talking to me, I mean, hearing her say the kind of things that she'd say. Always steady. Always supportive. Always encouraging, telling me it was OK, everything would be OK. ''You'll see''. How many times did she say that.' She took a deep breath and breathed out slowly.

'Sounds like it was also important what she said to you as well.'

Mandy nodded. 'She was steady. I mean, that's kind of a strange thing to say about your Gran, but she was. I mean, it was chaos at home. I mean, well, yeah, it was. Just how it was. Nothing ever seemed organised. But with Gran, I mean, it was different. I liked that.'

'You liked how it was, without the chaos.'

'She did things at particular times. She watched particular TV programmes. She had her routines, stuff like that. And, well, you kind of knew what she'd be doing at particular times on particular days. I'd go around and I'd know when she'd be having tea, you know. At home, well, you never quite knew, meals happened when they happened. But with Gran that wasn't how it was.'

'Sounds like meal times with Gran sort of stand out?' Ian wondered whether he was putting meaning into Mandy's comment that was not there, but then it was something she had highlighted and chosen to communicate. He just noticed his slight concern and let it go to keep his focus on what happened next.

'She'd cook herself. It wasn't always out of a packet and into the microwave.' Mandy felt that discomfort arising within herself. She wasn't sure she wanted to talk about food. She wasn't sure how Ian was going to react. She shuffled awkwardly in the chair. Ian noticed the somewhat forced movement, or so it seemed to him. Food. He made the recognition to himself and accepted that this was going to be a sensitive topic, and that he needed to be sure that his empathy was utterly reflective of his client, no agenda, no getting ahead, and that there was total acceptance of whatever Mandy sought to communicate.

'Yeah, sounds like she cooked her own things, things she made?'

Mandy nodded. 'Yeah.' She didn't want to talk about it, and yet somehow, somewhere deep inside herself was this urge to talk. And she felt emotional, and she didn't know why. Her eyes suddenly filled with water. She blinked and turned away, feeling suddenly hot. She closed her eyes, seeking to regain her composure. 'But that was then, that was how it was.' She sought to put the memories aside.

'That was how it was then with your Gran. Good times, huh?'

Yes, Mandy thought, they were good times. But . . . The thought flooded into her brain, how could they be? How could she have eaten so many different things, and enjoyed it? And then it all stopped and she only had home food, and school. Yuck. She felt suddenly silent inside. She was confused. It wasn't that she had specific thoughts. She simply didn't know what to think. The discomfort began to appear again inside her. She sighed.

'Difficult memories?'

She shook her head. 'It's just so confusing. I don't know what . . .' She shook her head.

'Confused by it all, just don't know what . . .', Ian shrugged, trying to convey his understanding of that sense of not knowing.

Mandy knew that her Gran would probably be like everyone else, now, encouraging her to eat. And she found that hard to accept or acknowledge. She didn't want to think about it but it kept coming back at her, and had done during the week. But she could hear her voice in her head, telling her to just eat something. She didn't want to hear her voice, but she did as well. She wanted to talk to her Gran, and she wanted to hear her voice, but she didn't want to hear her telling her that. She wished she could say it, she wanted to say it, but she was afraid. She didn't know what Ian would say. She wasn't aware that she was rubbing her hands together again.

Ian could see the hand movements, but he had also seen a change in Mandy's expression. She looked anxious, her jaw looked tight, her eyes were staring in a different way.

'You look anxious, Mandy, I'm here if you want to tell me, but I respect your choice if you'd rather not.' He felt utterly sincere in what he had said.

An example, perhaps, of where the tone is more important than the words, the sincerity in the way the counsellor speaks is more therapeutic than what he is actually saying.

Mandy heard the sincerity in his voice, but she still wasn't sure. Her heart was thumping and her head felt a bit weird. 'You want me to eat, don't you?' She wasn't sure quite why she had asked the question but it sort of blurted out. But she looked at him and waited for his reply.

'I want to help you to resolve what's eating you on the inside, Mandy.' Ian maintained eye contact. The words were a genuine expression of what he was feeling, what he was experiencing.

Genuineness, authenticity, transparency – the counsellor is conveying what he is experiencing, and doing so without hesitation. Yes, the words may seem loaded, but sometimes the counsellor has to trust the direct nature of what emerges within them. Trusting one's process as a counsellor is important. Within the therapeutic encounter what is vital is that in any moment when a counsellor expresses what he or she is experiencing they must be sure that they are to some degree integrated into the relationship with the client. In other words, if the counsellor is not significantly in contact with the client (and there will be a debate as to just how much is necessary on the continuum of contact) then it is likely that what comes to mind for them is less likely to have relevance to the client, and arguably should not be communicated. The counsellor who thinks they are being person-centred because they tell the client what they experience, regardless of the degree and nature of the contact and integration into the relationship, is a menace and is not person-centred. Congruence is not permission to say anything simply because you experience it when you are in the room with a client.

Ian looked so serious, so caring, as Mandy continued to look at him. He knew his use of words might not have been helpful, he didn't know, but those were the words that came to him in the moment and he voiced them, trusting his own process to direct him to say what was needed. He felt integrated into the relationship with Mandy, he felt a sense of connection. He waited. Mandy looked away.

'She'd be telling me to eat.' Mandy spoke quietly, almost as though she didn't really want Ian to hear, and maybe because she didn't want to hear her words herself. But they had been spoken, and they had been heard, by both of them.

'Your Gran would tell you to eat?'

Mandy nodded. 'But she doesn't know what it's like.'

'No, she doesn't know what you know.'

'You said you didn't think I was fat.'

Ian nodded.

'Why did you say that?'

'I was being honest with you.'

'I was looking at photos of myself when I was a child, with Gran. I looked sort of chubby, but I looked happy. I always seemed to be smiling.'

Ian nodded, 'lots of photos of a chubby you smiling with your Gran.'

'Mum says I don't smile any more.'

'That how it feels?'

Mandy shrugged. She guessed that her mum was probably right but didn't like to admit it, not to her mum anyway.

'Hard to accept?'

Mandy stuck her bottom lip out, and nodded.

'It's mean when parents are right and you don't want to admit it.'

Mandy nodded.

She hated being at home, hated how it was, how it made her feel. She wanted to get away. She sat silently with her thoughts. Ian respected the silence and allowed Mandy to continue to be with whatever she was experiencing in herself. 'But I am fat.'

Ian nodded. 'What can I say?'

'You still don't think so, do you?'

Ian shook his head. 'No. No, I don't.' This time he didn't qualify it as he had done previously.

The tone has changed. The difference of view is now being experienced differently by the client. Mandy is now hearing Ian, and something inside her is resonating to his view. She doesn't want to hear it, it contradicts what she knows to be true. And yet . . . she is anxious. She is vulnerable. This a necessary condition for constructive personality change. It is vital that the counsellor maintains the therapeutic conditions. Ian is being genuine with Mandy. Mandy is now struggling to be genuine within herself. She doesn't know what to believe, not necessarily because it is Ian who is saying something different, but because somewhere inside herself there is beginning to stir a sense that he may be right. It may be very small, but it will hear what Ian has said, enabling Mandy to hear, in a way that previously she couldn't and didn't want to.

Mandy felt wretched inside, utterly confused and unsure of herself, and not at all sure how she had got to where she was in herself. She looked down, not knowing what to say or think. She felt tired, tired of it all, tired of everything. 'I don't understand . . .'

'Can you say what it is you don't understand, Mandy?'

'I'm fat. I feel it, I can see it. No one believes me.'

'Yeah, that sounds like an awful place to be, knowing something but no one else believes you.' Ian sought to warmly yet gently empathise with the dilemma. Mandy was speaking quite differently. This wasn't the hard, defensive Mandy that he had experienced before. She was much more reflective, trying to make sense of a fundamental contradiction, trying to make sense of it rather than just dismissing what everyone else thought. Ian knew this was a critical phase and he wasn't going to disturb what was happening for Mandy.

Mandy took a deep breath. 'I'm tired. I don't understand.'

'Must wear you out and, yeah, hard to make sense of.'

Mandy looked up suddenly. 'Is there something wrong with me?' Mandy needed to ask the question but she didn't want to as well. She didn't want to maybe hear that there was something wrong with her, but if there was nothing wrong why did it all feel so wrong, so confusing. Why? *WHY?* The question screamed in her head.

'Does it feel like there is something wrong?'

'Something's not right. I mean, if I'm thinking I'm fat but I'm not . . . , but I am, I know I am, I *know* I am.'

Ian nodded, 'yes, I know that you know you are, Mandy, and I'm not going to question that.'

'If my Gran was here she'd say it was OK, and probably tell me to eat something, and I probably would. I mean, that's how it was. I always did when I was with her. But since she's been gone, I mean, I don't know, it's all different.' Mandy was quite animated as she spoke. The anxiety was clearly present in her voice.

'Yeah, it's all become different since she's been gone.'

Mandy lapsed back into silence. Ian felt his heart going out to her, so much to have to cope with and yet he also wanted to acknowledge the presence of the actualising tendency which would be working to bring something constructive out of this experience if he could continue to maintain the therapeutic conditions. He just knew how important it was. He could feel tears in his own eyes momentarily and a rush of goosebumps. Come on Mandy, he could feel the words in his head, you're edging closer.

Ian is being human. These thoughts can arise. And it can be so easy to want to nudge the client along, but that's not what will be helpful. The client has to be allowed to process what is happening at their own pace. Ian is right to keep his thoughts to himself. But he is touched, he is affected, and he should be. The client is edging closer and closer to seeing things differently and of course that's going to have an impact on him. The person-centred counsellor acknowledges what they are experiencing. They may not communicate

> it in words, but perhaps it is communicated in some way into the relational atmosphere simply because it is present for the counsellor and the counsellor has a psychological contact with the client.

Mandy felt more and more tired. She could hardly keep her eyes open. 'Sorry, I can't keep awake.'

'That's OK. You've been through, are going through, a lot. It burns up energy. You need to look after yourself.'

'Can I go?'

Ian nodded. 'Sure. But look after yourself, Mandy. You're going through a lot at the moment.'

> Is part of Mandy inducing tiredness to block the therapeutic process? It could be. It happens. The anorexic part of herself is now under threat and will seek to assert control. The counsellor does not react by trying to stop Mandy going. He accepts what she says, what her needs are as she is experiencing them in the moment, but he does convey his hope that she will look after herself. He is conveying unconditional positive regard. The part of her that wants to block the process may therefore feel accepted. It quietens down. She stays a bit longer and the therapeutic exchange continues.

Mandy nodded. 'You seem to sort of understand.'

'I try my best.'

Mandy smiled. 'Am I wrong?' She frowned, shaking her head as she asked the question.

'No. You experience what you experience.'

> A counsellor might say, 'yes, you are wrong', but Ian hasn't. He's stayed with what Mandy believes. It's enough that she is now just voicing the question, 'am I wrong?' He is not exerting any pressure, if anything he is standing back and allowing her space in her dilemma.

'But . . .' Mandy paused, 'but, oh I don't know. I don't know.'

'No, take your time.'

'I keep thinking of those photos, of me and Gran, of me, smiling.' Mandy shook her head. 'It's not like she's me, I mean like I'm not her any more, or something like that. I don't know. It's hard to explain, but it's like I know she's me, but she isn't. And I don't know who I am . . . I don't know who I am.'

'Like waking up and not knowing who you are.' Ian wasn't sure whether he'd been helpful. He just had this sense of Mandy waking up from ..., not a dream, but a something and finding nothing was quite how she thought it was, and that wasn't right, because that was too dramatic ... or was it? He didn't know. He'd said what he'd said, unsure whether it was helpful. Maybe he should have just reflected back Mandy's words.

Mandy decided she needed to leave. She sort of wanted to go, but didn't. It sort of felt suddenly safe being here in the counselling room with Ian. Out there it seemed too busy, too many people in her life. She needed time, time to think. 'I think I need to go. I need time on my own to think.'

'Sure. Take care of yourself and if it feels difficult, is there anyone you can talk to?'

Mandy shook her head. 'Maybe I could try talking to mum a bit, maybe. She'd be OK with me talking about Gran.'

'Gran was your mum's mum?'

Mandy nodded.

Ian smiled. 'You both lost someone special?'

Mandy nodded. 'Yeah, I'll try. Maybe.' She wasn't sure, but felt that maybe she could, maybe, at the right time and if dad wasn't around. Maybe.

Mandy leaves but she is leaving from a different place in herself to where she was a few minutes before. Now she is more reflective. She is not reacting, her leaving is not driven by the part of her that is under threat. She's leaving in a more controlled way, with a purpose. She needs time to think, her own time, her own space. And Ian is not in any way blocking that. Again, he is conveying warmth, expressing concern that she look after herself. He's not telling her what to think, he's not trying to intervene in what she feels she needs to do. It's an important interaction. And it's hugely validating for Mandy to feel she can make her own choice, and it is a choice emerging from that part of her that is able to contain the idea that maybe, just maybe, she's wrong, or at least, she needs to hear what others are saying and maybe deep inside her what she is saying.

Mandy headed off home leaving Ian to be aware of just how drained he was feeling after the session. He knew he felt concern for Mandy, her world was in a sense breaking up, at least the way she saw things. It seemed that she was now beginning to be able to at least acknowledge a place for self-questioning. How she would be as a result, he did not know. But he did know that a battle was going to rage within her, and he hoped that she would speak to her mother and that she would be supportive in some way. It felt like if Mandy got more people still telling her to eat, it might drive her back into that anorexic side of her nature. She didn't need that. And he appreciated that people were concerned and were acting in a way that they felt were in Mandy's best interests. And they were right. She probably did need to eat more. But she needed to, what had he said, resolve what was eating her on the inside first.

Points for discussion

- How are you feeling? How are you dealing with those feelings? What would you do to regain your focus had you been Ian in this session?
- What were the critical moments in this session, and why?
- Reflect on the session and the process in terms of person-centred theory. How would you present this session in a case study?
- How do you feel Ian's practice may have been affected by his previous supervision session?
- What would you take to supervision from this session?
- Write notes for this session.

CHAPTER 11

Counselling session 7: 'I'll try – that's all I can say, I'll try'

The session had begun with Mandy saying a little about her week. 'I talked to mum, asked her whether she missed Gran, and said that I did and that I'd been talking about her to you. It actually helped a little. I seemed a little, I don't know, it just seemed to go OK.'

'Mhmm, so, talking to your mum seemed to go OK.'

'I still miss Gran, but somehow I feel a bit different after last week. I've got to accept it, haven't I? And I was thinking as well, I mean, I do want to get away from home and, well, maybe going to University would be good for that. Maybe. Saw my doctor again, though, talked to me about my Average Expected Body Weight – that was what he called it, based on my size and age, I think he said, not sure about that. But, anyway, he said I was getting too low and he weighed me and showed me a chart. He'd done this before but, well, I never really paid much attention before. But this was different. I guess I was different. Maybe I listened more, I don't know. I'm confused. I told him that I didn't feel underweight, and he asked how I was getting on seeing you. I told him it was OK, that I had got upset talking about Gran, but that it was good to have someone to talk to about things.'

'Seems like it was a different experience, you reacted differently.'

'I still didn't want to hear what he was saying, but I sort of found myself listening more, you know. But I still don't really understand. I mean, OK, I think I can see what he's saying, but it's not how I feel about myself, and that's what's real to me.'

'What's reality to you is different to what he's telling you.'

Mandy nodded. 'And that's confusing me. I don't understand. He tried to explain about how people can feel things about themselves that are distortions. But it doesn't feel like that, it really doesn't.' Her voice became higher pitched as she completed what she was saying. She shook her head and lapsed into silence, slumping back into the chair and looking suddenly very miserable and lost. 'I know I'm fat, I want to believe there's something wrong with what he's telling me, it doesn't make sense. It just doesn't.'

'No, that's what makes it so difficult, it doesn't fit with what you are experiencing and have been experiencing.'

'He said people do experience this, talked about how girls look at magazines and want to be like these slim models and sort of idealise some kind of image of themselves, that was how he put it. Yeah, I mean, I look at the pictures and, yeah, 'course I want to be like them, and I want to get into you know, clothes like other girls do. And I do, and I want to be slimmer.' She pinched her side. 'Look, that's fat, I don't want it.'

To Ian what Mandy had pinched seemed minute, but, OK, she had managed to pinch some flesh through her blouse. 'That feels like fat to you?'

'Well, isn't it?'

'If that wasn't there, what would be there?'

'Well, nothing, my ribs, I suppose.'

'And I guess that's how you want to be, so you can feel your bones through your skin?'

Ian wasn't at all sure that he was responding anything like a person-centred counsellor, and yet he also felt that he needed to be genuine here with how he was responding in himself to what Mandy was saying.

What is happening here? It feels as though both client and counsellor are interacting differently. There's a different tone. Mandy's saying it as it is for her, and Ian's being quite provocative in his response. He's pushing, gently, but he's pushing. Maybe appropriately given the tone of the exchange. Maybe the physical nature of what is being talked about has somehow made the exchange more solid in some way, more tangible. But is what he is saying therapeutically helpful? It seems to be. Can this process, this inter-action be trusted as therapeutic?

It feels like there is a mutual respect that has developed between Mandy and Ian. She's able to say what she feels but is able to hear what Ian is saying. He feels more able to be more direct in his responses and feels that Mandy is able to handle this without reacting against it. The relationship has shifted. But there will be a limit to what is happening and a point will come when there will need to be a moving on. But it seems that Mandy has moved to more of an acceptance of the need to agree to differ as opposed to fight against it. It means that she has moved to feel able to some degree accept that there is another view to her own. She's not going to accept that the other view is right, not yet, maybe she never will, but she can now toler-ate the existence of this other view.

'No, I mean, well, I don't know. But if I can't feel my bones then I'm fat, aren't I?'

'So what you are saying is, maybe I'm wrong, but what you seem to be saying is that if you feel anything between your ribs and your skin, then that's fat and you have to get rid of it?'

Mandy nodded.

'So does that mean muscles, flesh, anything that gets in the way has to go?'

'But it doesn't feel right.'

'No, and I do hear what you are saying Mandy, that anything that gives you a feeling of some kind of bulk between your skin and your ribs feels like fat, makes you feel fat.'

Mandy nodded. 'The doctor told me that I needed to put on weight, but that would mean, you know', she pinched her sides.

'Yeah, it would.'

Mandy took a deep breath. She felt confused still. It was like being told one thing that sort of seemed reasonable but it didn't fit with what she knew. And she didn't know what was right. She knew what felt right. She knew she felt fat, she knew it. And yet . . . And that was the problem. And she felt quite energised by what had just been discussed. She felt like she was, yeah, fighting her corner, but it was different. She was listening, not just blocking what others said. 'You think I should put on weight?'

'What can I say, Mandy. If your Average Expected Body Weight is low, well, it does indicate that you need to put on weight, and, you know, I can hear you struggling with the feeling that that doesn't feel right, that you don't want to feel more weight on your body.'

'I see lots of girls, they look like me, I don't suppose they're all being told to eat more.'

'Mhmm, there are lots of girls like you, but I don't know what they're being told.'

'I can't put on weight, it won't feel right.'

'No, it won't. You experience yourself as being fat and the thought of eating more and putting on more weight is unacceptable, yes?'

Mandy nodded. 'And I know Gran would have told me to eat, I know she would have done. She always talked about having regular meals. I used to like visiting her and having tea with her.'

Ian nodded, 'something to enjoy, having tea with Gran'.

'Oh, I don't know. I'm still confused. It's like everyone else sees something that I don't.'

'Yeah, and the way you see it is important to you.'

Mandy nodded. 'I don't have many things I can control in my life, but, well, what I eat, I can control that.'

The counsellor has stepped back. He is acknowledging how it is for Mandy. She has now acknowledged her need for control and the role of eating in that process.

'And it seems that you do that really well.' Ian smiled.

'I suppose I do, don't I?' Mandy smiled back. And then the smile faded, almost as soon as it had appeared. Her thoughts suddenly went back to the photos and she heard herself asking a question. It was a question she was asking herself but she was actually voicing as well. 'What happened to the little girl who smiled?'

'What did happen to her, Mandy?' Ian spoke softly, sensing the fragility of the process and not wanting to in anyway disturb it.

> The relational tone has changed quickly and the counsellor has had to be sensitive and responsive to this. Suddenly something very significant has been said, packed with emotion. From verbal jousting to smiles and warm appreciation for what Mandy is good at, and now the little girl who doesn't smile any more. Things can move fast when the client enters a state of psychological flux like this. The counsellor has to be focused, has to be. It's a crucial phase in the therapeutic process and in the therapeutic relationship. Can the counsellor stay with Mandy as she experiences her own internal emotional roller-coaster? He has to. However hard it might be for him, it is harder for her.

'She lost her Gran, she lost her reason to smile, she felt very small in a big world.'

Ian nodded, 'she lost so much and it left her feeling so small.'

Mandy stayed silent. There was nothing to say all of a sudden. She sat, staring down, wondering, where was the little girl that smiled? Where was she? Where was *she?*

Ian didn't say anything. He let the silence be. He didn't know what Mandy was experiencing but he trusted that whatever it was was timely and necessary. He didn't need to know what it was.

Mandy continued to sit in silence. It wasn't just the photos. She had memories. Sitting at the table at Gran's. Being given a slice of chocolate cake. Part of her wanted to smile, she knew that she would have been smiling, but her lips remained tightly shut. She couldn't smile. She wanted to smile, but she couldn't.

Mandy sighed heavily. Her shoulders were stiff. She was sitting stiffly. She tried to relax. It all seemed such a struggle. 'What do I do?'

'What do you want to do?'

'Smile, have things to smile about. But I have to keep in control, you know?'

'Mhmm, control's important, yeah.'

Mandy nodded her head, and then stopped. 'But I can't, can I, I mean, not really. Things happen. Don't they? I mean, I can't stop myself growing up, not really.'

'You've tried to.'

Mandy nodded, 'I know. But ...' She shook her head again. 'I'm wrong aren't I, somehow. I'm wrong. But how could I be? But I am. And yet it doesn't make sense, not really. I know what the doctor told me, told me that what I was experiencing wasn't unusual, that it happened and it took a while to think differently, and that I had to try. But I don't know how to.'

'Mhmm, hard to imagine how to think differently.'

'And I already am, aren't I, a bit? I mean, I wasn't thinking like this when I first saw you.'

'No, no, you weren't. You weren't thinking like this at all.'

'Hmm. But it won't feel right, I know it won't. Just thinking about putting on weight, feeling bigger, I mean, it won't feel right, it won't be me.'

'No, it won't feel like the you that you are used to feeling.'

Mandy stared down at the floor suddenly feeling very unsure of herself. She knew that her Gran would want her to eat, but she wasn't sure if that was what she wanted. She didn't know what she wanted. She didn't know who to listen to. Everyone telling her what to do, well, almost everyone. That was what made the counselling different. She kind of knew that Ian wanted her to eat. He didn't say so directly, but, well, she sort of sensed it. But at least he'd been honest, and said that he did appreciate that she felt differently. And that was important, someone who sort of understood that she really did feel fat. And her doctor had been better with her that last time. Or had she just listened to him that time? What was going on? She didn't understand. She wanted someone to tell her what to do, what was right, what was best. She wanted her Gran. And yet she knew what her Gran would say. It felt like she had to eat a little more, somehow, somehow, however wrong it felt. But that just felt impossible.

'You look really thoughtful, Mandy. A lot to make sense of.'

'I need to eat more, don't I, even though I don't feel like it.'

'That's how it is, yeah?'

'That is what I have to do, don't I?'

Ian could feel the pressure to confirm what Mandy was saying. Would he be simply introducing an external locus of evaluation? Maybe. But Mandy had said that she needed to eat more, he would simply be agreeing with her, not telling her what to do. That felt OK. It felt honest, genuine. He nodded. 'I think so.'

Mandy sighed. She knew he was right even though she felt it was wrong. It was like being split in half. 'I'll try. That's all I can say. I'll try.'

'You don't need to say any more. To say "I'll try" is a big enough change, yes?'

Mandy nodded. 'The doctor talked about anorexia, but that happens to other people, you know, and I don't want to accept that. Maybe I've got a problem, maybe, but I don't want to think of myself like that.'

'No, you don't want to think of yourself like that.'

'I've just got to learn to try and eat a little more and, what, do I keep seeing you?'

'Sure, if you want, if you feel it would be helpful to come and talk about things.'

'Yeah.' Mandy paused. 'It's so hard to imagine.'

'Hard to imagine . . . ?'

'Eating more, and the thought of putting on weight. The doctor wants me to come in regularly so they can monitor it, see the nurse. That's what I have to do, isn't it?'

'You think it will help?'

'Maybe. Maybe. It feels so much, too much. I still feel like I'm trying to make sense of it.'

'Mhmm, a lot to make sense of, and you need time for that.'

'Yes. Would you talk to the doctor, tell him that? I feel I'll get rushed and I couldn't cope with that.'

'Sure, I can let him know. Slowly build yourself up and adjust to it, and keep talking about whatever . . .'

Mandy nodded.

The session continued with Mandy reflecting on how difficult it all was, how hard it was to accept, that she didn't want to accept it and yet she also felt she had to. It felt very intense once again and by the end of the session Ian was feeling drained, and so was Mandy. Mandy had decided she needed to talk some more to her mother, explain how she would try to put on a little more weight, but how hard it was, and to take it slowly. She felt her mum would listen, particularly after they'd talked the previous week about Gran. She felt things were easier there for her. And Ian agreed that she could use the counselling sessions to talk about how things were going, but also talk about anything else that was coming up for her. They had no set limit on the number of sessions, it would take as long as it took, but for Ian, and for Mandy, a turning point had been reached. Inwardly, Mandy was changing, and with this was the hope that any change in her eating behaviour would be underpinned by her feeling different about herself, her life, her future and her past.

It is three weeks later. Mandy is persevering. She missed one session, she was finding it all too difficult. She has arrived for the tenth session feeling distressed. The session has already begun.

Counselling session 10: who am I now?

'It's not easy, I'm finding it so hard. Everything in me just recoils from eating. And yet, I know I have to, I feel more certain about that. It's like people seem to be putting less pressure on me to eat and it's making it easier, somehow. But I need their encouragement as well.' Mandy was looking at Ian and feeling very uncertain. 'It's like I just don't know who I am anymore. I mean, I know who I am, but it's who I was. Not who I am. I feel so empty, like I don't exist, but I do.' She shook her head, feeling tearful once again.

'And it's so distressing not having a sense of who you are.'

Mandy nodded, unable to hold back the tears any more. 'I didn't expect this, and it would be so much simpler to just not eat again and be the me that I was. I hate all this.'

Ian felt for her, the pain and the struggle on her face. 'Yes, so much to hate about what's happening for you.'

'I just want to feel OK. I felt OK before, now, well, now I don't, and everyone tells me that I look better, but I don't feel better. Will I ever feel OK?'

'You wonder if you'll ever feel OK again, yes, and it doesn't help people telling you that you look better when you don't feel better.'

'Mum does that. I know she means well, I do, but I react. It makes it harder, it really does. I wish someone would talk to her.'

'You'd like someone to talk to her?'

'Someone who could explain how difficult it is. I tell her but she only sort of hears, but then she forgets, I suppose, and starts to push me. I know she wants to help, but she gives me too much food. She's too positive, cheery, and I don't need that.'

'You need her to be different, not so pushy?'

Mandy nodded. 'I wish you could talk to her, make her understand.'

'You'd like me to talk to her, make her understand how it is for you?'

'I wish you would. Would you? Do you do that sort of thing?'

'I'd be happy to, but I wouldn't talk about you and what you've told me. But I could say something about the difficulties and what you feel is going to be help-ful. Or, you could tell her and I could be here to support you as you tell her?'

'She sort of takes over a bit.'

'What would you like to do?'

'If she could maybe come along at the start of a session, maybe, ten minutes, that would be good.'

'OK, you talk to your mum and see if she can come, what, next time?'

Mandy nodded.

'OK. And it's about things that you want your mum to understand, yes?'

Mandy nodded.

'OK.'

The session moved on. Mandy felt relieved although a little tense as well wonder-ing how her mother would be, and how it would feel having her in the counsel-ling room. She returned to talking about how hard it was to know who she was.

'It's like I've sort of woken up from a kind of dream, but it's more than a dream, I mean, it's real, it's what's been happening, and in a way I haven't really woken up, it's like I'm sort of still in the dream as well.' She shook her head.

'Yes, like you're still living in the dream but trying to be awake as well.'

'And I don't know if I'm the person in the dream or the person trying to be awake.'

Ian nodded, 'mhmm, am I the person in the dream or the person who's trying to wake up?'

'I sort of hadn't realised it would be like this. I mean, it's not like you can just forget about everything and just, well, be different. It's like I sort of stopped, somehow, part of me still feels sort of like I was when I was 15.'

'When your Gran died?'

Mandy nodded. 'And that's not really clear either. I mean, yes, I do feel like I did, sort of, and then I don't as well.'

'You do feel like you did and you don't, as well. And it's not clear, sounds really confusing.'

Mandy was nodding. 'It is. I'm sort of focusing on school a lot, I mean I sort of use that in a way to, I don't know, gives me a focus. Or I listen to CDs and stuff, but it's like I don't know what to listen to. I sort of want to listen to stuff from a few years back, but also stuff from now as well. It's like I sort of like different things but sometimes I feel I don't like it.'

Ian nodded. His sense was that Mandy was experiencing herself in parts, and that each part – some being linked to periods in her life which in turn connected to her eating control – had its own preferences. He knew she had gone through an intense set of experiences, and she had probably generated configurations within her structure of self, some of which may feel quite differentiated. She was an amalgamation of them, plus whatever that was emerging now.

'You sort of change, feel different at different times.'

'Can't seem to settle.' She frowned. 'Is it always like this?'

'Can be. Different parts of you.'

'That's how it feels. I really feel like I just want to blow it all away, but I can't and if I did, there'd be nothing left. That's how it feels, sometimes, when I get down, I don't know who I am, and it can feel, I don't know. Just down.'

'Yeah, you feel down and it's something about there being nothing there. Is that what you mean?'

Mandy nodded. 'I slip into thinking about not eating.' She rubbed her face. I can lose myself, and then I sort of come out of it. But when I come out of it it's like, well, yeah, you know, it's like the dream's more real than waking up.'

'Mhmm, the dream, how you feel when you think about not eating, that feels more real.'

'And shouldn't the dream feel less real? It all feels back to front and I don't know. What do I do? Just keep trying?'

'It takes time. You've been so much one part of you that it's really difficult to break out of it.'

'It feels like that. Like being trapped, but you sort of know what it's like being trapped. When you're free it's weird.'

Ian nodded and thought about people in prison, or people held in solitary confinement for long periods of time. In a way Mandy had been locked away inside herself, or inside part of herself, he wasn't sure how best to describe it. Part of her seemed right.

'Like you're trapped somewhere.'

'I wish it would all just . . . , go away.'

'You'd like to feel free of it all?'

'I spend time in my room, thinking and then trying not to think. I don't want to think about anything.'

'You don't want to think about anything, you just want to stop thinking?'

'My brain wants to explode sometimes, it feels like, yeah, it wants to explode. I want to empty it out, you know, but then, well, yeah, start again maybe . . . Maybe.' Mandy went quiet. She knew that then she'd be facing that nothingness and she hated that as well. It just made her feel so tired. She yawned.

'Yeah, makes you feel tired, huh?'

Mandy nodded. 'And that's another thing. I never used to feel so tired. I mean, I sort of did more recently, but I didn't use to.'

'Mhmm, more tired at the moment than you're used to.'

'I mean, you know, months back I wasn't so tired. Before I started seeing you, yeah, that's when I started to feel tired.'

'That's when the tiredness began.'

'It feels worse now. Still, be Easter soon, no school, but then there's exams next term.'

'So, bit of a break but work to do as well.'

The session continued with Mandy talking again about how difficult it all seemed, and Ian trying to ensure that she felt heard and understood. Mandy talked about how she hoped to do well in her exams, and at least be in a position to think about university, though she wasn't sure what she wanted to do. She was able to acknowledge that at least she had a chance now of thinking about what she wanted, but she felt like she needed to keep her options open, but that felt hard, that she sort of wanted to know what she was doing.

The session ended with Mandy going back to the idea of her mum coming to the next session – she felt apprehensive but it also felt right as well. Ian gave her time to explore what it felt like, what her hopes and concerns were, and this helped. Mandy left feeling good that it had been her idea and that Ian had taken her seriously. She just hoped her mum would listen to what Ian had to say.

Points for discussion

- How would you describe Ian's style of working as a person-centred counsellor? What are his strengths? What are his weaknesses?
- Describe the changes in Mandy. Relate these changes to Rogers' Seven Stages of Constructive Personality Change.
- How might you have responded differently in these two sessions had you been Mandy's counsellor?
- What is your reaction to the idea of Mandy's mum attending the start of the next session? What opportunities and difficulties do you foresee in this?
- What would you anticipate to be the major difficulties that Mandy will face over the coming weeks, months, in fact years, as she seeks to move on from her anorexia? What do you feel will be most helpful in helping her?
- What would you take to supervision from this session?
- Write notes for this session.

Reflections

Ian's reflections – 'For me the supervision session was actually really important in the way it enabled me to strengthen my own belief in the actualising tendency and in the way that I work. I do feel good that Mandy is now able to question her beliefs about herself. It's an awful process, your whole sense of self is brought into question, and it cannot be rushed, it has to take place at a pace that the person's structure of self can cope with. Too much, too quickly can be shattering. It's bad enough when it is taken slowly.

'I am aware of just how powerful the sessions have been for me. I am left not knowing quite what to say. I was asked to comment on what felt most significant. Saying about what was eating at Mandy on the inside, that seemed significant. Seemed to contribute to moving the process on. It was something that was sort of drawn out of me. I sometimes wonder whether the actualising tendency in the counsellor conspires with the actualising tendency in the client in some way, drawing out of the therapist responses that are right and timely, though they may seem inappropriate to the outsider. I think this is an area we don't understand too well. Something about intuition in that as well. But I am moving away from the point.

'And having to respond to her direct questions. I admire her for asking me so directly. She must have hoped, at first, I'd take her side, and when I didn't, well, I knew that it was a kind of moment of truth in the therapeutic relationship. But we continued, and somehow I think it proved to be helpful. We knew where we stood. Nothing was hidden. That has to be good for the therapeutic process.

'I am so glad that I have time to work with Mandy and I'm not only able to offer "time-limited" counselling. I know from other clients that they prefer seeing someone in the surgery and don't want to have to be referred off somewhere else. It can take time to form a therapeutic relationship and yet the building of that relationship is part of that therapeutic process. Why am I saying that? Well, it feels important for people to have time to do this, particularly where the issue or issues are deep-seated or are major factors that have contributed to that person's structure of self.

'It's not easy for Mandy. She really is now encountering herself beyond her "anorexic self", and I'm not sure I like to use that term, but, well, it seems to sum the situation up. She's finding it desperately difficult to know who she is. The way she has seen herself over the past four years has become steadily more ingrained. The need for earlier recognition and response to these kinds of conditions is so apparent. There needs to be so much more education in recognising signs of difficulty and how risk and damage might be minimised. It was a good idea for her mother to come along. It was Mandy's idea. She was feeling frustrated in one session at not feeling able to communicate what it was like to her mum. She asked if her mum could see me. I agreed though made it clear that it would be an information session and that I wouldn't be disclosing anything about what Mandy had been telling me. It went well. Where a young person feels this is likely to be helpful, well, I think it can be a good idea. But I wouldn't suggest it, it would have to be something that the client suggests or wants.

'So, I hope Mandy continues to attend. I hope that by offering her person-centred counselling she will find her way through the changes that are happening within her. Is it hope? No, it's more than that. I know that she will find her way, what I don't know is what form that way will take, and what changes of behaviour may emerge out of changes in herself. But that's the challenge and the joy of working this way, being part of a therapeutic process in which you see a person becoming . . . No, I'm not going to say what they become, that will emerge as it emerges, when it emerges, and cannot be predicted.'

Mandy's reflections – 'He's quite cool, you know. Didn't think that way when he said he didn't think I was fat. Bastard. But, yeah, he's OK. He listens. He's like my Gran, well, in some ways. It's good, but it's not easy. Still not really getting my head round it all, but I'm trying and, as time goes on, more and more is making sense. I'm eating more now, and have started to put on a bit of weight. I don't like it, feels weird, but people are encouraging me, but not pushing me too much. I'm up to my sixteenth session now. It's been hard, and I've really questioned whether it's all worth it. But, well, people have encouraged me, not pushed me too much and Ian's given me time to talk and make sense of who I am and who I want to be.

'So, yeah, never thought I'd end up seeing a counsellor. But it's helped me. It's good to be listened to, to feel that someone's trying to understand it the way you see it. You don't get that very much. Most people want to give you their opinion all the time, tell you what's best for you. Sometimes they're right, but sometimes they just don't understand.

'Don't know what else to say. Oh, I've decided to go to university. Not sure yet what I really want to do, but that's me, still trying to work out who I am and what I want. But I think it'll be good for me. I'm not going to one too far away. Home's sort of become more important. I think because things are better between me and mum. She's being great. She came and had a chat with Ian as well, something I suggested. I sort of wanted her to hear from someone how difficult it all could be. I think that helped a lot.

'What now? I don't know. I sort of take life one day at a time. Starting to think differently and feel different, but it's slow. I know I need to get out more, meet people, stop spending so much time dwelling on myself. I think I'd like to do something environmental. I've joined a local group. Try and sort out the mess the adults have made of the world. Got to sort myself out first, though, but I'm getting there.'

Author's epilogue

It's taken a while to write this book, I felt really stuck writing the second scenario. It was only after I attended a wonderful play called 'Over the Edge' about working with young people with psychosis and the importance of early intervention that I got an idea as to how to develop it. Not that anorexia is a psychotic state. But it could be for some people, depending on what drives them into self-starvation.

I hope the two scenarios presented in this book have been helpful in enabling you to engage with the process and enter into the hearts and minds of the clients, counsellors and supervisors. The scenarios by no means cover all the many facets of working with women who are experiencing bulimic and anorexic states. Such conditions develop for so many different reasons and each client must be worked with as a unique human-being, even though their behaviours may be similar. The behaviour is an outer symptom of an inner condition – unique to that person – and this itself exists in response to sets of experiences which themselves are unique to that person.

As usual, I am left wondering how Carol and Mandy will fare in the years ahead. I know they are fictitious characters, and yet they do become alive, at least to me and I hope to you. Will Carol contain her urge to binge and move away from having to think about managing that urge? Will she be able to become a woman no longer hampered by the damaging impact of Tommy on her life? And how will her relationship with her parents develop in the years ahead? And what of Mandy? Still in those early weeks of change. Still coming to terms with the contradictions within herself, and the struggle to find herself, become herself, pick up the threads, perhaps, from before those anorexic years? Does it work like that? Can we really set aside experiences? Maybe we can work on their effects but the memories will remain to some degree, but maybe they will no longer trigger unwanted behaviours.

Eating is such a fundamental aspect of the human experience. It is a behaviour through which we express ourselves. 'We are what we eat', some will say, and maybe it is equally true to say that we 'eat what we are'. What we choose to eat reflects something of our own priorities, our own sensitivities, and certainly our own preferences.

Dukler and Slade (1988) make the important point concerning how much a person suffering from anorexia/bulimia can construct their sense of self around food and body control, and that even when a change in their eating pattern is made, this underlying reality can and often does remain. They make the point that in terms of therapy, 'for the anorexic nervosa/bulimia sufferer . . . [t]he task is not to assist her in enhancing the self she has. It is the more delicate process of enabling her to create and define herself anew' (p. 203). There is often a sense of 'who am I?', of not knowing, nothingness, behind the body-control, eating/starvation-centred sense of self that has come to dominate the person. This reality must be heard, warmly accepted and empathised with by the person-centred therapist. Slowly, gently, painfully, the client is encouraged – by the presence of the therapeutic conditions – to develop and establish a fresh sense of self. It cannot be rushed or forced. The person-centred counsellor is offering the relational climate within which the client can begin to tentatively become a new person, or should we rather say claim a fresh-sense of personhood.

I do believe that the person-centred approach has so much to offer this client group, and I wish to return to the notions of 'constructive personality change' and 'constructive behaviour change'. The link between these two and the way the person-centred practitioner works with the client seems to be significant. The person-centred counsellor or therapist offers a set of therapeutic conditions knowing that their presence facilitates 'constructive personality change'. This, then, impacts on the internal processes that drive a person, or should we say encourage a person, to follow certain patterns of thought and behaviour. It seems to me that sustainable change requires us to go beneath the cognitive and the behavioural, to engage with the person, to form a relationship with that person that encompasses as much of that person's personhood as they are able to bring into the counselling process.

For me, person-centred is exactly what it says it is, a process in which the person of the client is the primary focus for the work. It is not behaviour-centred, or centred in any specific area of the person, but the whole person. If clients are to develop the positive self-regard referred to in this book as an essential part of their process of constructive personality change then they have to feel and experience the core conditions of the person-centred approach, they have to feel unconditional positive regard, experience empathic understanding and know that the person they are with is being authentically present in the relationship.

I hope this book, at least in part, provides a basis for readers to explore further what the person-centred approach has to offer women with eating disorders.

Appendix

Rogers' seven stages of constructive personality change

Stage 1

There is an unwillingness to communicate self. Communication is only about externals.

Feelings and personal meaning are neither recognized nor owned.

Personal constructs are extremely rigid.

Close and communicative relationships are construed as dangerous.

No problems are recognized or perceived at this stage.

There is no desire to change.

There is much blockage to internal communication.

Stage 2

Expression begins to flow in regard to non-self topics.

Problems are perceived as external to self.

There is no sense of personal responsibility in problems.

Feelings are described as unowned, or sometimes as past objects.

Feelings may be exhibited, but are not recognized as such, or owned.

Experiencing is bound by the structure of the past.

Personal constructs are rigid, and unrecognized as being constructs, but are thought of as facts.

Differentiation of personal meanings and feelings is very limited and global.

Contradictions may be expressed, but with little recognition of them as contradictions.

Stage 3

There is a freer flow of expression about the self as an object.

There is also expression about self-related experiences as objects.

There is also expression about the self as a reflected object, existing primarily in others.

There is much expression about or description of feelings and personal meanings not now present.

There is very little acceptance of feelings. For the most part feelings are revealed as something shameful, bad, or abnormal, or unacceptable in other ways.

Feelings are exhibited, and then sometimes recognised as feelings.

Experiencing is described as in the past, or as somewhat remote from self.

Personal constructs are rigid, but may be recognized as constructs, not external facts.

Differentiation of feelings and meanings is slightly sharper, less global, than in previous stages.

There is a recognition of contradictions in experience.

Personal choices are often seen as ineffective.

Stage 4

The client describes more intense feelings of the 'not-now-present' variety.

Feelings are described as objects in the present.

Occasionally feelings are expressed in the present, sometimes breaking through almost against the client's wishes.

There is a tendency toward experiencing feelings in the immediate present, and there is distrust and fear of this possibility.

There is little open acceptance of feelings, though some acceptance is exhibited.

Experiencing is less bound by the structure of the past, is less remote, and may occasionally occur with little postponement.

There is a loosening of the way experience is construed. There are some discoveries of personal constructs; there is the definite recognition of these as constructs; and there is a beginning questioning of their validity.

There is an increasing differentiation of feelings, constructs, personal meanings, with some tendency toward seeking exactness of symbolization.

There is a realisation of concern about contradictions and incongruences between experience and self.

There are feelings of self responsibility in problems, though such feelings vacillate.

Stage 5

Feelings are expressed freely in the present.

Feelings are very close to being fully experienced. They 'bubble up', 'seep through', in spite of the fear and distrust which the client feels at experiencing them with fullness and immediacy.

There is a beginning tendency to realize that experiencing a feeling involves a direct referent.

There is a surprise and fright, rarely pleasure, at the feelings which 'bubble through'.

There is an increasing ownership of self feelings, and a desire to be these, to be the 'real me'.

Experiencing is loosened, no longer remote, and frequently occurs with little postponement.

The ways in which experience is construed are much loosened. There are many fresh discoveries of personal constructs as constructs, and a critical examination and questioning of these.

There is a strong and evident tendency toward exactness in differentiation of feelings and meanings.

There is an increasingly clear facing of contradictions and incongruences in experience.

There is an increasing quality of acceptance or self-responsibility for the problems being faced, and a concern as to how he has contributed. There are increasingly freer dialogues within the self, an improvement in and reduced blockage of internal communication.

Stage 6

A feeling which has previously been 'stuck', has been inhibited in its process quality, is experienced with immediacy now.

A feeling flows to its full results.

A present feeling is directly experienced with immediacy and richness.

This immediacy of experiencing, and the feeling which constitutes its content, are accepted. This is something which is, not something to be denied, feared, struggled against.

There is a quality of living subjectively in the experience, not feeling about it.

Self as an object tends to disappear.

Experiencing, at this stage, takes on a real process quality.

Another characteristic of this stage of process is the physiological loosening which accompanies it.

The incongruence between experiences and awareness is vividly experienced as it disappears into congruence.

The relevant personal construct is dissolved in this experiencing moment, and the client feels cut loose from his previously stabilized framework.

The moment of full experiencing becomes a clear and definite referent.

Differentiation of experiencing is sharp and basic.

In this stage, there are no longer 'problems', external or internal. The client is living, subjectively, a phase of his problem. It is not an object.

Stage 7

New feelings are experienced with immediacy and richness of detail, both in the therapeutic relationship and outside.

The experiencing of such feelings is used as a clear referent.

There is a growing and continuing sense of acceptant ownership of these changing feelings, a basic trust in his own process.

Experiencing has lost almost completely its structure-bound aspects and becomes process experiencing – that is, the situation is experienced and interpreted in its newness, not as the past.

The self becomes increasingly simply the subjective and reflexive awareness of experiencing. The self is much less frequently a perceived object, and much more frequently something confidently felt in process.

Personal constructs are tentatively reformulated, to be validated against further experience, but even then, to be held loosely.

Internal communication is clear, with feelings and symbols well matched, and fresh terms for new feelings.

There is the experiencing of effective choice and new ways of being (Rogers, 1967, pp. 132–55).

References

Bentall RP (1990) The syndromes and symptoms of psychosis. In: RR Bentall (ed.) *Reconstructing Schizophrenia*. Routledge, London.

Bozarth J (1998) *Person-Centred Therapy: a revolutionary paradigm*. PCCS Books, Ross-on-Wye.

Bozarth J (2001) A reconception of the necessary and sufficient conditions for therapeutic personality change. In: J Bozarth and P Wilkins (eds) *Rogers' Therapeutic Conditions: evolution, theory and practice*. Volume 3: *Congruence*. PCCS Books, Ross-on-Wye.

Bozarth J (2002) Empirically supported treatments: epitome of the specificity myth. In: JC Watson, RN Goldman and MS Warner (eds) *Client-centred and Experiential Psychotherapy in the 21st Century: advances in theory, research and practice*. PCCS Books, Ross-on-Wye, pp. 168–81.

Bozarth J and Wilkins P (eds) (2001) *Rogers' Therapeutic Conditions: evolution, theory and practice*. Volume 3: *Congruence*. PCCS Books, Ross-on-Wye.

Bryant-Jefferies R (2001) *Counselling the Person Beyond the Alcohol Problem*. Jessica Kingsley Publishers, London.

Bryant-Jefferies R (2003) *Time Limited Therapy in Primary Care: person-centred dialogues*. Radcliffe Medical Press, Oxford.

DiClemente CC (2003) *Addiction and Change*. The Guildford Press, New York.

DiClemente CC and Prochaska JO (1998) Towards a comprehensive, transtheoretical model of change: stages of change and addictive behaviours. In: W Miller and N Heather (eds) *Treating Addictive Behaviours* (2e). Plenum Press, New York.

Dukler M and Slade R (1988) *Anorexia Nervosa and Bulimia*. Open University Press, Buckingham.

Embleton Tudor L, Keemar K, Tudor K *et al.* (2004) *The Person-Centered Approach: a contemporary introduction*. Palgrave MacMillan, Basingstoke.

Evans R (1975) *Carl Rogers: the man and his ideas*. Dutton and Co., New York.

Gaylin N (2001) *Family, Self and Psychotherapy: a person-centred perspective*. PCCS Books, Ross-on-Wye.

Gilbert S (2000) *Counselling for Eating Disorders*. Sage, London.

Hallam RS (1983) Agoraphobia: deconstructing a clinical syndrome. *Bulletin of the British Psychological Society*. **36**: 337–40.

Hallam RS (1989) Classification and research into panic. In: R Baker and M McFadyen (eds) *Panic Disorder*. Wiley, Chichester.

Hallett R (1990) Melancholia and Depression: a brief history and analysis of contemporary confusions. Unpublished Masters Thesis, University of East London, London.

Haugh S and Merry T (eds) (2001) *Rogers' Therapeutic Conditions: evolution, theory and practice.* Volume 2: *Empathy.* PCCS Books, Ross-on-Wye.

Kirschenbaum H (2005) The current status of Carl Rogers and the person-centred approach. *Psychotherapy.* **42**(1): 37–51.

Kutchins H and Kirk S (1997) *Making us crazy: DSM: the psychiatric bible and the creation of mental disorders.* The Free Press/Simon Schuster, New York.

Marchant L (2005) From private correspondence.

Mearns D and Thorne B (1988) *Person-Centred Counselling in Action.* Sage, London.

Mearns D and Thorne B (1999) *Person-Centred Counselling in Action* (2e). Sage, London.

Mearns D and Thorne B (2000) *Person-Centred Therapy Today.* Sage, London.

Merry T (2001) Congruence and the supervision of client-centred therapists. In: G Wyatt (ed.) *Rogers' Therapeutic Conditions: evolution, theory and practice.* Volume 1: *Congruence.* PCCS Books, Ross-on-Wye, pp. 174–83.

Merry T (2002) *Learning and Being in Person-Centred Counselling* (2e). PCCS Books, Ross-on-Wye.

Orbach S (1979) *Fat is a Feminist Issue . . .* Hamlyn Paperbacks, London. (Originally published in 1978 by Paddington Press Ltd.)

Patterson (2000) *Understanding Psychotherapy: fifty years of client-centred theory and practice.* PCCS Books, Ross-on-Wye.

Prochaska JO and DiClemente CC (1982) Transtheoretical therapy: towards a more integrative model of change. *Psychotherapy: theory, research and practice.* **19**: 276–88.

Rogers CR (1946) Significant aspects of client-centred therapy. *American Journal of Psychology.* **1**: 415–22.

Rogers CR (1951) *Client-Centred Therapy.* Constable, London.

Rogers CR (1957) The necessary and sufficient conditions of therapeutic personality change. *Journal of Consulting Psychology.* **21**: 95–103.

Rogers CR (1959) A theory of therapy, personality and interpersonal relationships as developed in the client-centred framework. In: S Koch (ed.) *Psychology: a study of a science.* Volume 3: *Formulations of the Person and the Social Context.* McGraw-Hill, New York, pp. 185–246.

Rogers CR (1967) *On Becoming a Person.* Constable, London.

Rogers CR (1980) *A Way of Being.* Houghton-Mifflin Co., Boston, MA.

Rogers CR (1986) A client-centered/person-centered approach to therapy. In: I Kutash and A Wolfe (eds) *Psychotherapists' Casebook.* Jossey Bass, New York, pp. 236–57.

Russell GFM (1979) Bulimia nervosa: an ominous variant of anorexia nervosa. *Psychological Medicine.* **9**: 429–88.

Slade PD and Cooper R (1979) Some difficulties with the term 'schizophrenia': an alternative model. *British Journal of Social and Clinical Psychology.* **18**: 309–17.

Sharman K (2004) From compliance to concordance: a psychological approach to weight management. *Healthcare Counselling and Psychotherapy Journal.* **12**: 111–22.

Thompson C (1996) Older Women and Eating Disorders. http://www.mirror-mirror.org/edwom.htm

Tudor K and Worrall M (2004) *Freedom to Practise: person-centred approaches to supervision.* PCCS Books, Ross-on-Wye.

Vincent S (2005) *Being Empathic: a companion for counsellors and therapists.* Radcliffe Publishing, Oxford.

Warner M (2002) Psychological contact, meaningful process and human nature. In: G Wyatt and P Sanders (eds) *Rogers' Therapeutic Conditions: evolution, theory and practice.* Volume 4: *Contact and Perception.* PCCS Books, Ross-on-Wye, pp. 76–95.

Weiner M (1989) Psychopathology reconsidered: depression interpreted as psychosocial interactions. *Clinical Psychology Review.* **9**: 295–321.

Wilkins P (2003) *Person-Centred Therapy in Focus.* Sage, London.

Wilkins P and Bozarth J (1998) Unconditional positive regard in context. In: J Bozarth and P Wilkins (eds) *Rogers' Therapeutic Conditions: evolution, theory and practice.* Volume 3: *Unconditional Positive Regard.* PCCS Books, Ross-on-Wye, pp. vii–xiv.

Wyatt G (ed.) (2001) *Rogers' Therapeutic Conditions: evolution, theory and practice.* Volume 1: *Congruence.* PCCS Books, Ross-on-Wye.

Wyatt G and Sanders P (eds) (2002) *Rogers' Therapeutic Conditions: evolution, theory and practice.* Volume 4: *Contact and Perception.* PCCS Books, Ross-on-Wye.

Useful contacts

Person-centred

British Association for the Development of the Person-Centred Approach (ADPCA)
Email: adpca-web@signs.portents.com
Website: www.adpca.org

An international association, with members in 27 countries, for those interested in the development of client-centred therapy and the person-centred approach.

British Association for the Person-Centred Approach (BAPCA)
Bm-BAPCA
London WC1N 3XX
Tel: 01989 770948
Email: info@bapca.org.uk
Website: www.bapca.org.uk

National association promoting the person-centred approach. Publishes a regular newsletter *Person-to-Person*.

Person-Centred Therapy Scotland
Tel: 0870 7650871
Email: info@pctscotland.co.uk
Website: www.pctscotland.co.uk

An association of person-centred therapists in Scotland which offers training and networking opportunities to members, with the aim of fostering high standards of professional practice.

World Association for Person-Centered and Experiential Psychotherapy and Counselling
Email: secretariat@pce-world.org
Website: www.pce-world.org

An association that aims to provide a worldwide forum for those professionals in science and practice who are committed to, and embody in their work, the theoretical principles of the person-centred approach first postulated by Carl Rogers. The association publishes *Person-centred and Experiential Psychotherapies*, an international journal which 'creates a dialogue among different parts of the person-centred/experiential therapy tradition, supporting, informing and challenging academics and practitioners with the aim of the development of these approaches in a broad professional, scientific and political context'.

Problem eating issues

American Anorexia/Bulimia Association
Website: www.aabainc-org

Eating Disorders Association
103 Prince of Wales Road
Norwich
Norfolk NR1 1DW
Helpline tel: 0845 634 1414
Email: helpmail@edauk.com
Website: www.edauk.com

Invisible
Maureen Schiller Consultancy
18 Kings Road
Chalfont St Giles
Buckinghamshire HP8 4HS
Email: invisible@maureenschiller.co.uk

'Invisible' is a highly innovative multimedia resource that makes eating disorders and the underlying issues visible, with editions for individual (parents, young people, anyone interested in health and well-being) and professional (school nurses, teachers, PSHA co-ordinators, youth workers, health visitors, counsellors, CAMHS professionals) use.

National Association of Anorexia and Associated Disorders
Website: www.anad.org

National Centre for Eating Disorders
54 New Road
Esher
Surrey KT10 9NU
Tel: 01372 469493
Website: www.eating-disorders.org.uk

National Obesity Forum
PO Box 6625
Nottingham NG2 5PA

Tel: 0115 8462109
Website: www.nationalobesityforum.org.uk

Overeaters Anonymous
PO Box 19
Stretford
Manchester M32 9EB
Tel: 07000 784985
Email: info@oa.org
Website: www.oagb.org.uk

The British Dietetic Association
For practical advice about healthy eating visit its consumer website.
Website: www.bdaweightwise.com

The Obesity Awareness & Solutions Trust (TOAST)
Latton Bush Centre
Southern Way
Harlow CM18 7BL
Tel: 01279 866010
Email: enquiries@toast-uk.org.uk
Website: www.toast-uk.org.uk

Index